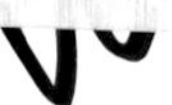

Triathlon. The Mental Battle

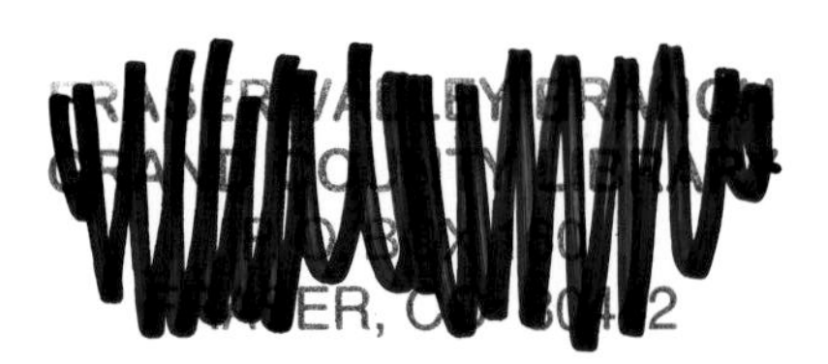

Mark Kleanthous

Triathlon. The Mental Battle

How to be a Better Athlete by Taking Control of Your Mind

Meyer & Meyer Sport

British Library Cataloguing in Publication Data
A catalogue record for this book is available from the British Library

Triathlon. The Mental Battle
Maidenhead: Meyer & Meyer Sport (UK) Ltd.,
ISBN: 978-1-78255-026-6

Aachen, Auckland, Beirut, Budapest, Cairo, Cape Town, Dubai,
Hägendorf, Indianapolis, Singapore, Sydney, Tehran, Wien

Member of the World Sport Publishers' Association (WSPA)

Printed by: B.O.S.S Druck und Medien GmbH, Germany
ISBN: 978-1-78255-026-6
E-Mail: info@m-m-sports.com
www.m-m-sports.com

Dedicated to my wife Clare for putting up with the clicking of my keyboard late into the evening and walking up to more clicking early in the morning. I proved anything is possible if you put your mind to it.

Thank you to everyone who took part in answering my many questions to help with writing this book.

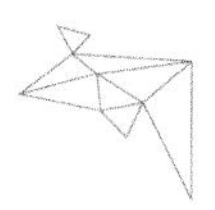

„It's not the mountains that we conquer but ourselves."
Sir Edmund Hillary

TABLE OF CONTENTS

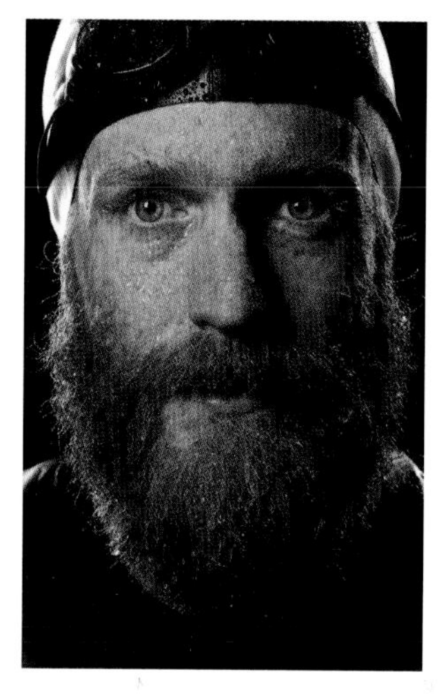

FOREWORD

By Sean Conway

It is unlikely that anyone else in the world has competed triathlons for 32 consecutive seasons—Mark Kleanthous is that person.

He has crossed the finish line in more than 460 triathlons including 36 Ironman® distance events, 2 double Ironman® distance events and a triple Ironman® distance event.

In all the events he has started, he has finished with the exception of two; his two DNFs—Did Not Finish—one due to being hit by a car, the other being hit by a tree!

Through his vast experience, Mark Kleanthous has learnt and developed the most effective coping strategies to overcome the fears that we all have, whether we are embarking on our very first competition or aiming to complete an event of extreme endurance. He has an attention to detail and a knowledge of preparation that is unsurpassed.

Mark has not only excelled in his own feats of endurance but he has helped and advised many athletes achieve their true potential and taught them how to overcome their doubts and trepidation for over the last 20 years.

In this book, you will learn how to overcome your natural fears, learn how to take control of your mind and take your body where it has never been before.

You will learn to control your emotions so your personal feat is an achievement of joy and true satisfaction rather than one of stress and dread.

This book can make all the difference between achieving your ambition with control and calm and being comotosed with the fear of failure.

This book is a must read for every person considering a triathlon or wanting to improve their sporting performance.

Mark believed in me and he has helped me achieve my latest endurance event when others thought it was not possible.

Sean Conway

First & only person in history to swim the length of Britain—Land's End to John O'Groats (900+ miles)

Round the world cyclist

http://www.seanconway.com/

@Conway_Sean

INTRODUCTION

This book explains how to prepare mentally for triathlons and endurance multi-sport events. Once you consider taking part in competing, you increase the risk of mental melt down. This book will help you develop an automatic response mechanism to deal with doubts and fears. The book is not about mental toughness but learning how to train the mind.

Triathlons are physically demanding, which is why many people compete in endurance events. The harder it is to prepare for and complete a triathlon, the greater the sense of achievement.

Many triathletes train 10 hours a week or more, and long distance athletes may devote 600 hours preparing over many months. Despite spending a lot of time training, the majority of triathletes' concerns were not about training but the mass swim start, environmental factors, mechanical failure, nutrition and hydration. Few spent much more than 1% of their training time preparing mentally.

Most people think about what they are going to say in everyday life.

This could be a job interview, work meeting, meeting someone for the first time for a date, important telephone conversation or making a complaint. If you are running late for a meeting or competition, the best way is to mentally get yourself ready. Actresses and actors go through their mind time and time again thinking about how they will act before every performance. People who don't prepare often reflect on "what if" after the event. You should use this mental strategy for triathlon. In this frenetic world we live in with limited time to train, mental rehearsal is something we should all practice.

Almost all of the athletes that compete to the best of their ability prepare by mentally rehearsing. Part of moving from choking to being a champion is in the mind. Most of the leading athletes in the world also use a mental coach at least once in their careers while many use them all the time.

Mentoring and positive thinking are not just for elite professional athletes; they should be used by everyone. We have all witnessed one athlete beating another by the tiniest of margins. Often the runner-up looked the best or was the favorite. What separated the performance was what the person was thinking.

Because every second counts, mental rehearsal can be the difference between choking due to mistakes and being a champion.

The reason I believe that some people do not need to repeat an action 10,000 times or need to practice 10,000 hours to achieve excellence is because of mental visualization.

Training often can have no purpose, but practicing is more specific and improves weakness and strengths.

I have known athletes suffer a debilitating injury that has forced them to stop practicing, but mentally visualize only to gain better skill coordination when they resume training.

Time by itself does not lead to greatness; if it did then the person who trained the most would be world and Olympic champion.

In his 2008 bestseller, Outliers, Malcolm Gladwell wrote about the 10,000-hour rule. One factor that allows people to achieve proficiency that is as good if not better than a professional is putting in 10,000 hours of practice or work toward a goal.

His findings make common sense—if someone spends 10,000 appropriately coached hours, they could obtain greatness.

However, you simply do not achieve your ultimate skill, fitness or performance when you get to 10,001 hours of preparation.

Proficiency at most things takes more than just practice time. Some people achieve greatness in 5 years, many achieve it in 10 years, while some people take 20 years.

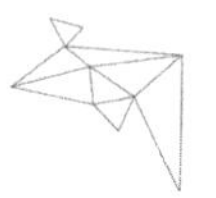

> **"I've missed more than 9000 shots in my career. I've lost almost 300 games. 26 times, I've been trusted to take the game winning shot and missed. I've failed over and over and over again in my life. And that is why I succeed."** Michael Jordan

Natural ability by itself is no guarantee of success.

There are many roads to greatness, but logging 10,000 hours of practice on its own to help perfect a skill is not sufficient.

Delving into the mind with positive mental rehearsals can help an athlete that chokes and underachieves improve considerably.

Use accurate training diaries (using heart rate monitors), recording every second minute hour percentages in each heart rate zone.

Maybe comparing thousands of athletes training files will one day in the future lead to a more accurate conclusion on how to achieve greatness.

Expert performances are often based on the athlete being able to focus on the sport at that time and ignoring thoughts about other things.

Kaufman's research found that practice accounted for more than 4 times as much variance as the amount of working memory. So practice is important but accounted for 30% variance in excellence. He believes that everyone can be a genius at something but not everything.

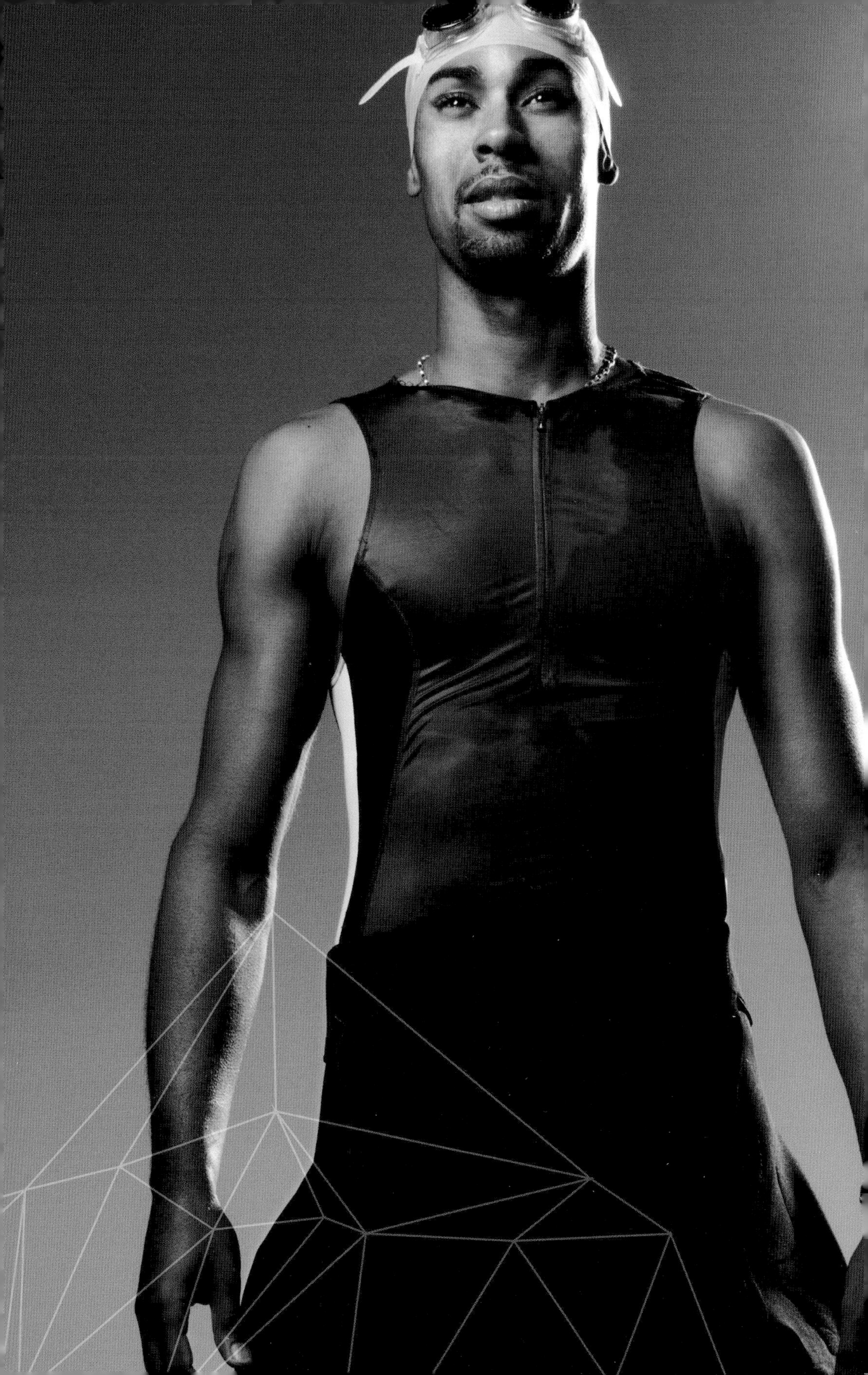

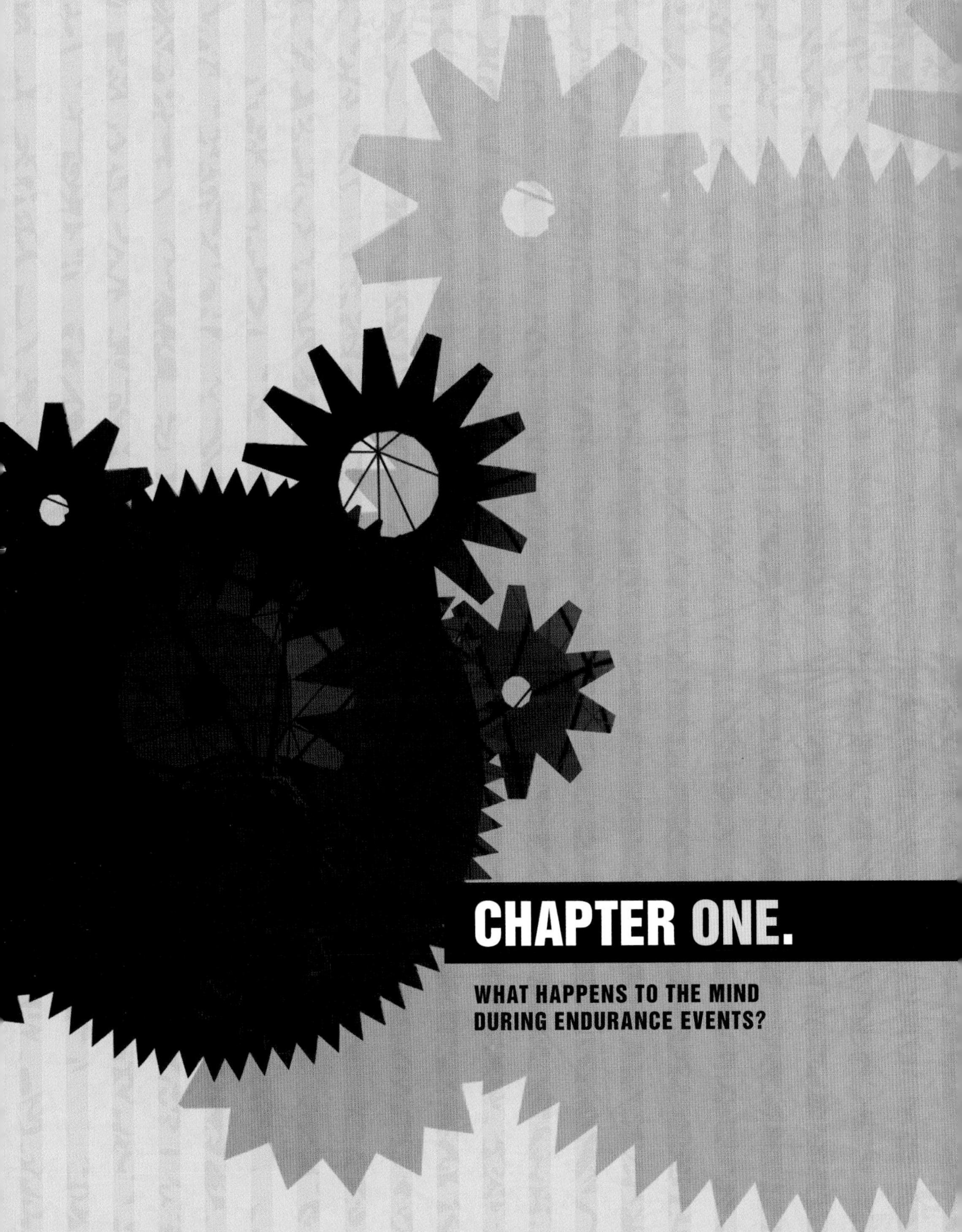

CHAPTER ONE.

WHAT HAPPENS TO THE MIND DURING ENDURANCE EVENTS?

ONE.

WHAT HAPPENS TO THE MIND DURING ENDURANCE EVENTS?

Discomfort, pain and low energy are hurdles you must overcome to get to the finish line of a triathlon. Changing the way you think about obstacles can help you overcome them.

Thoughts in your mind should not be like driving down a one-way street or the motorway. Control your attitude by changing speed or slowing down your thoughts, as this will help you change your mind's direction.

"Negative self-talk"–this happens due to a distorted view on what is happening.

"All or nothing thinking"–this way of thinking is based on monitoring success or how you performed on the day based on current conditions and issues that may have happened.

"Catastrophizing"–expecting mistakes will happen or you are unlucky.

"Never satisfied"–this type of thinking is natural, and you will always find ways to keep improving even during a triathlon. If you fall behind on hydration, make sure you get back on track as soon as you can.

"Over-generalizing"–jumping to a conclusion, often based on emotion rather than facts. For example, I had a terrible triathlon before looking at the results to see the winner was 10 minutes slower than last year.

The subconscious mind controls our perception of pain. Make sure you expect to be in some discomfort; otherwise it will shock the mind when it happens.

Mental rehearsal is important. Remember when you first learned to drive or swim, there was so much to take in and process.

When I first learned to drive many years ago, my mind was full with changing gears, mirror signals, maneuvering, steering and braking, etc. I am far more vigilant now and aware of what is going on around me when I drive than when I was first learning.

I remember thinking, how will I remember to do all these things I needed to drive. I practiced taking many driving lessons, then took my test and failed. A few weeks later, with just a couple of extra lessons, I passed. The major difference was I visualized myself driving well and passing my test.

The first step to success is thinking about success! Do you know what it takes from thinking to doing? All it takes is a positive frame of mind. Negative thoughts simply hold you back instead of moving you forward.

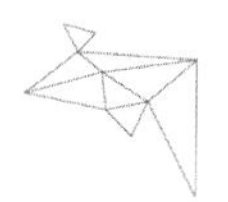

"Winners lose more times than losers, the more times you lose and learn the more times you win." Mark Kleanthous

With so much information now entering our minds every second of the minute of every day via the Internet, Facebook, Twitter, etc., it is increasingly more difficult to clear our minds to reboot and refresh. Today's modern frenetic lifestyles are increasing the amount of information our brains can cope with, almost to overloading proportions.

Clearing the mind takes practice, just a few minutes every day. It may take a week to have a totally clear mind just for a few minutes. In today's world of instant gratification, most people simply won't have the patience to reap the benefits. First you have to start by acknowledging a thought and letting it pass without clinging onto it.

Triathlon forums can be a wealth of information but can also cause confusion with many conflicting views of opinion. It is best to ask a qualified triathlon coach who has already experienced what you are trying to achieve. If you want opinions, ask lots of people; if you want advice, ask just one person who has experience and then trust your instincts.

The same goes for triathlon–the more things that you can learn the less your mind is busy. If you are competing in your first triathlon, or want to go faster next time then you need to visualize that you have no past experience. The busier your mind is the more chance you will find everything overwhelming, then negativity and doubt will soon follow.

A flitting mind will have lots of little thoughts and then will stop on a small, negative thought that will be magnified out of proportion. For example, during the triathlon, you might check your GPS watch and notice you are slowing down. Now you start to feel fatigue and then have more negative thoughts. However, in reality you were running up a slight uphill and had not noticed. A positive mind is often a quiet but alert mind, looking for results, while a negative mind is busy and looking for excuses.

A chattering mind is due to voices from your past, some are positive but we tend to wrecall the negative ones more often from our conscious. Make sure they do not cloud your mind unnecessarily. If we cling onto even the smallest of negative thoughts, we then blow them up out of proportion. You may drop a gel at a feed station and have many options–there are just a few below, but I am sure you can think of other options. This is exactly what I want you to do–decide now which the best action for you is.

1. Slow down or stop and get another thought.
2. Let this annoy you for the rest of the competition and potentially forget to catch up on lost calories.
3. Make sure you get a gel next time at the earliest opportunity; if not, slow down.
4. Check you don't have a spare with you, or in future always have a back-up plan.
5. Learn from your mistakes, be self-sufficient and carry all your nutrition.
6. Ask a competitor for an energy gel.

If you don't need a gel you could be giving your competitors the wrong impression and leading them into a false sense of security.

Most of my best performances and those of my athletes have been when the mind was quiet, and I let my subconscious get on with being competitive. This is known as the runner's high or "being in the zone." Thoughts in our minds while we are asleep can wake us up as nightmares; what was going on in the mind felt like reality. You can use your mind to overcome adversity and negativity and switch a negative to a positive. Fears, pain, negative thoughts and low moments in your triathlon can all be dealt with without any expense.

If you answer your own mind's question with a favorable response, this is usually enough to keep negativity from festering and growing into an imaginary major disaster waiting to happen.

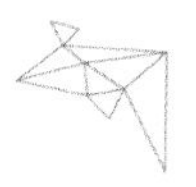

"In order to succeed, your desire for success should be greater than your fear of failure." Bill Cosby

For example, if you have concerns about the water temperature for your open water swim triathlon, instead of thinking, "I will be cold in my next open water swim," tell yourself a different way: "The water will be cold in my open water triathlon" as this helps you be more comfortable with your concern and makes it easier to believe your answer, "I have swum in colder water without a wetsuit, and it was OK."

It is amazing the water temperature will be the same on race day but your perception will not seem as bad.

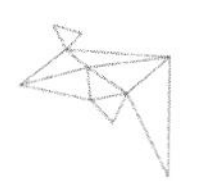

"It always seems impossible until it is done." Nelson Mandela

Change a negative into a positive. Challenge those perceptions of thought and who you think you are and switch them to who you want to be. Confidence comes from taking actions.

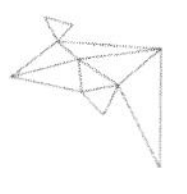

"Live as if you were to die tomorrow. Learn as if you were to live forever." Mahatma Ghandi

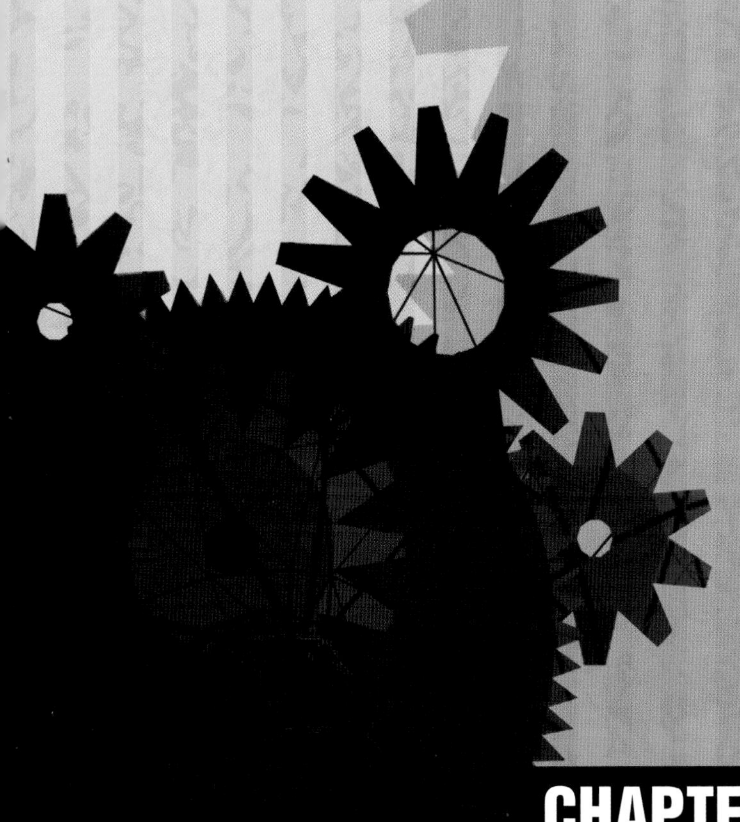

CHAPTER TWO.

PREPARING FOR TRIATHLONS

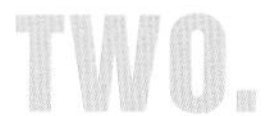

PREPARING FOR TRIATHLONS

The hardest part is probably starting to train for a triathlon. Generally, most people find that this is the exciting part of the journey. The next part can be fun, training and getting ready, with so many exciting sessions to complete to be race-day ready.

Then you are just weeks away from triathlon day. You have built up to the race and cannot think about anything else. You have great expectations until a week to go and now your thoughts easily wander thinking about all the things that can go wrong in the final week.

This is when people start to bite their nails and become moody. They don't sleep very well and can't think properly. I have even witnessed slurred speech from some very over-anxious triathletes up to 5 days before the start of the triathlon. These over-excited triathletes are suffocated by nerves.

Once the triathlon starts they often do not perform to the best of their ability, even though some of the anxiety has been defused from starting the race.

Here is what you can do to get race ready and not psyched out:

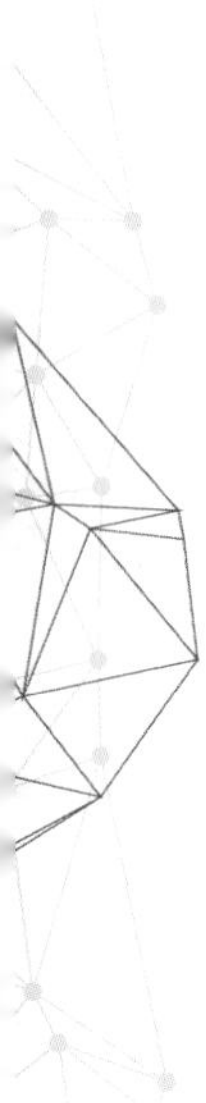

- Don't let the race-ready mind kill your performance.
- During the build-up, get excited not anxious.
- Avoid trembling in fear.
- Visualize a realistic, achievable challenge like making goals to push yourself, otherwise there is no point having something to work for.
- This could be to complete the triathlon without walking, targeting a particular time for one or all of the disciplines, finishing in time, going faster than previously or beating a competitor. Visualization is a necessary requirement for

your fundamental aspirations. If you do not think the whole dream through, it will cause you concerns, which leads to doubts.

- Putting your planned finishing time on your phone or as a reminder on your calendar or post-it notes can be a stimulus for some people but a big hindrance for others. Do what will help you stay focused and motivated, not things that create unnecessary stress.
- Use a mantra in training that you can use during the triathlon.
- During the taper period when you reduce the amount of training, spend the extra time repeating your mantra during visualization to help your confidence. If you fail to complete the image of yourself during the triathlon all the way through, expect anxiety to start increasing.
- Remember what training you have done and not the sessions you may not have been able to complete.
- Recall all the tough and great workouts you have completed.
- Remind yourself how unfit you were and how far you have progressed.
- Find inspiration from past sporting moments, such as from someone who has overcome adversity, a physically challenged triathlete, watch a triathlon DVD or be a spectator or even a volunteer. Read a few pages of a book at bedtime. Aim to finish it a few days before your triathlon as reading can help you unwind, allow your mind to relax, and help you sleep well.

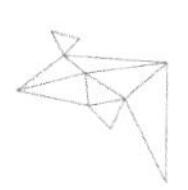

"There is only one thing that makes a dream impossible to achieve, the fear of failure." Paulo Coelho

DEVELOP A PLAN

Make a plan or list to help reduce anxiety, making sure that the plan is flexible and not so rigid that it gives you the jitters or makes you nervous.

Tri-check list—Create your triathlon checklist and tick off what you have and what you need. Can you find that lubrication for the swimming to avoid chaffing?

Tri-jobs list—Start arranging a "Things to do list." List anything that needs attention, such as extra cycle bottle cages that may need fitting or some extra spares fitted to your bike for racing.

Nutrition and hydration list and plan—Don't wait too late to get your favorite nutrition. Know when and where you are going to have it during the triathlon.

Travel arrangements—Have a plan for leaving home to get to the triathlon with adequate time.

Pace plan—By now you should know what condition you are in and what pace you can maintain. Think about the pace and know your race splits in order to keep yourself on track to avoid going too fast.

Race strategy—Make sure you know where to seed yourself for the swim, what order you will do things in the transition, what gearing to start the bike, how you will tackle the cycle section, and how you will pace the run.

Self-talk—Have different mantras for different parts of the triathlon day.

Pre-Script scrapbook—A lot of people complete a blog, post-race, but few athletes I know have a list of images and comments of what you want to happen. Either use images of yourself or positive images to create your own scrapbook. The whole experience can make you feel much more confident. This can be a physical example in an album or book, a set of images on your phone in chronological order, or a set of images in your mind.

Weather—You cannot control the weather. There is no such thing as bad weather if you have planned for all seasons. It's ok to check the short-range weather forecast but not every few hours unless a hurricane is coming!

Remind yourself you are doing a triathlon for fun, and you will enjoy it. You will then remain focused and strong and will have a great experience.

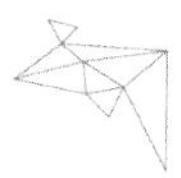

"Every thought we think is creating our future." Louise L. Hay

During a triathlon, you think things that cause nerves, anxiety, and fears:	Change this thought to:
"Another workout done and I am getting nervous–not long to go before my triathlon"	"Great workout, I am better prepared than yesterday."
"I will get knocked about in the swim"	"Take time to position myself for a great swim."
"I am getting very tired halfway through the run"	"Every step I take is one less to the finish line and less energy I need."
"I need to slow down or stop"	"I can recover and rest at the finish line."
"I am feeling uncomfortable"	"Get comfortable with feeling uncomfortable."
"My breathing is labored, I must give up"	"Keep going–that last heartbeat has sent more oxygen to my muscles."
"My leg is sore, I can't go on"	"Keep the pain under control; I can do it!"

Have a file in your mind for a better way of thinking and most importantly an answer for everything!

Most of all, you need to be adaptable to change your thoughts, dependable to rely on the positives and ignore negativity, be willing to learn from experience and be flexible on triathlon race day. Try to dream vivid images of positive visions to overcome negative thoughts.

Don't worry about how ridiculous your dream is, use it to outweigh the anxiety; don't forget both are fantasy. The strength of a dream will win 98% of the time over a weak conscious mind that creates fear. Let your mind win the battle before you do.

HABITS

If your confidence or concentration fades during a triathlon then, from personal coaching experience, it's because your mind is in control of your body instead of working in harmony. It is not because you are not mentally strong; it is because you simply did not train the mind.

Control the mind so it runs smoothly, and the muscles of your body will also work smoothly.

The Self-Sabotage Mind is a common problem when the pressure of head-to-head competition stress is not experienced in training. You need to train hard, and remember these sessions while you are doing them by filing them away for race day. A vast majority of athletes who never get beaten in training often choke on race day. The winners raise their performance level on race day, while the ones who are world-beaters in every workout simply cannot perform to the best of their ability.

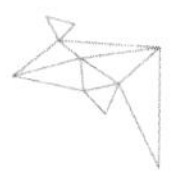

"Success is where preparation and opportunity meet." Bobby Unser

Every single triathlete can improve his performance by mentally rehearsing some negativity, then switching it by positive thinking.

Symptoms you are likely to experience without mental training:	How you will improve with mental training
Nervousness that builds from 48 hours to the start	Not nervous in the 2 days before the competition
Faster in training, slower in a triathlon	Faster in the triathlon with the same amount of training
Anxiety and fear become unbearable	Anxiety and fear are manageable
Injury before most competitions	No niggles, aches or pains in the build-up
Sickness before most competitions	Feeling strong and healthy in the build-up
Fitness drops before each triathlon	Fitness improves right up to the triathlon
Shaking on race morning	Small amount of trepidation
Unable to eat your normal breakfast race morning	Eat normal breakfast and digest it before the start
Unable to concentrate	Alert, aroused and ready to race but semirelaxed
Feeling sick in the stomach on race day	Looking forward to racing
Worrying about things that normally don't bother you	Nothing bothers you on race morning
Concerned about what others are thinking	Focusing on yourself
Inconsistent with race results	Consistent with race results as expected
Overly worrying about the „uncontrollables"	Confident to control any problems that may happen

POSITIVE SELF-IMAGERY

You need to have made in your mind a video "The Most Successful Triathlon Ever!" or whatever you want to call it. You have the leading role.

- Rehearse your video at every opportunity
- Try it during an easy workout.
- Progress to seeing it during a tough workout.
- Relax in a chair before you go to sleep.
- You need a quiet mind, so avoid being too relaxed and not too tired. Once you are competent then visualize it during a stressful situation and use the mind video to help you relax.

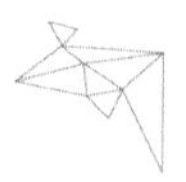

"A creative man is motivated by the desire to achieve, not by the desire to beat others." Ayn Rand

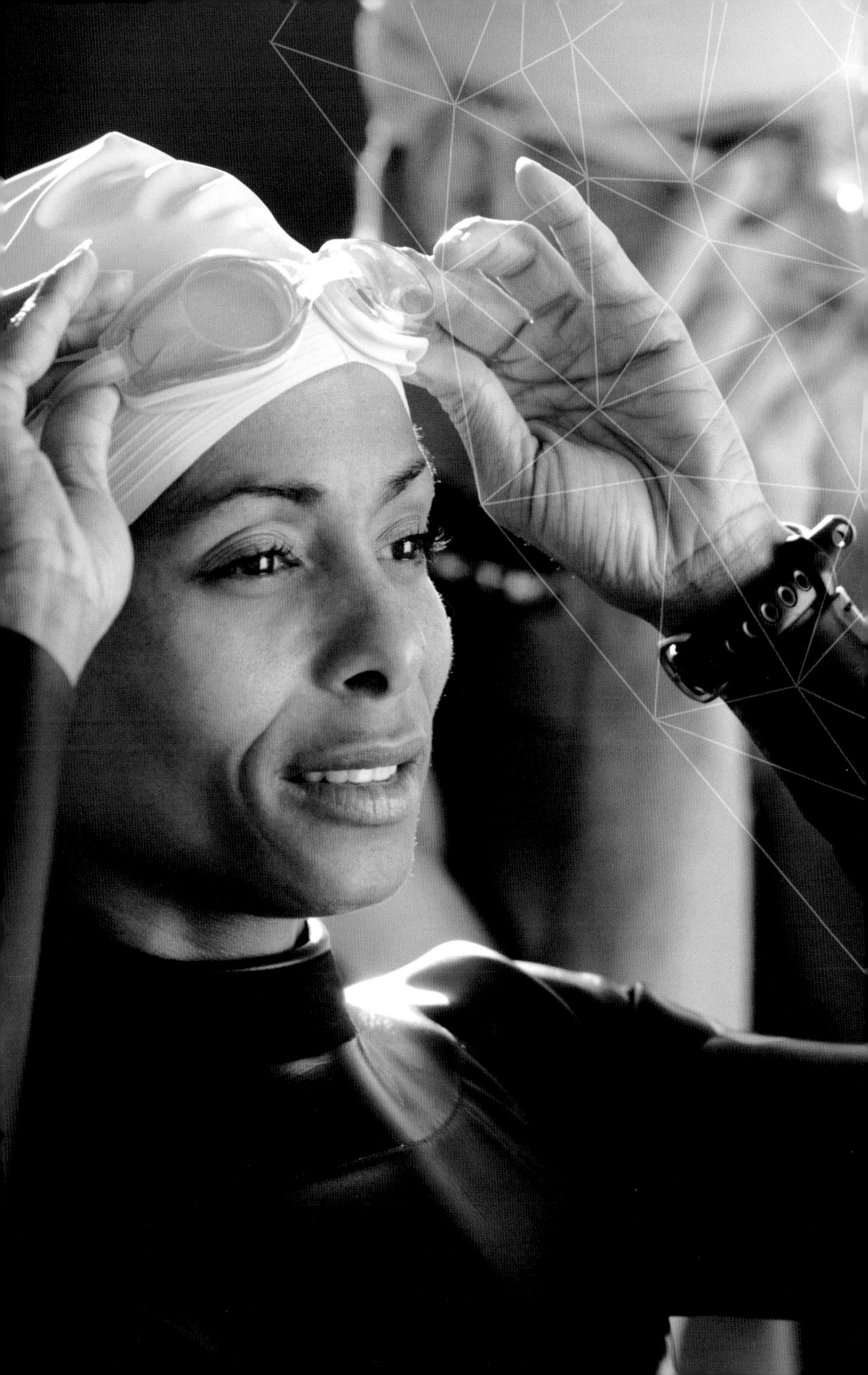

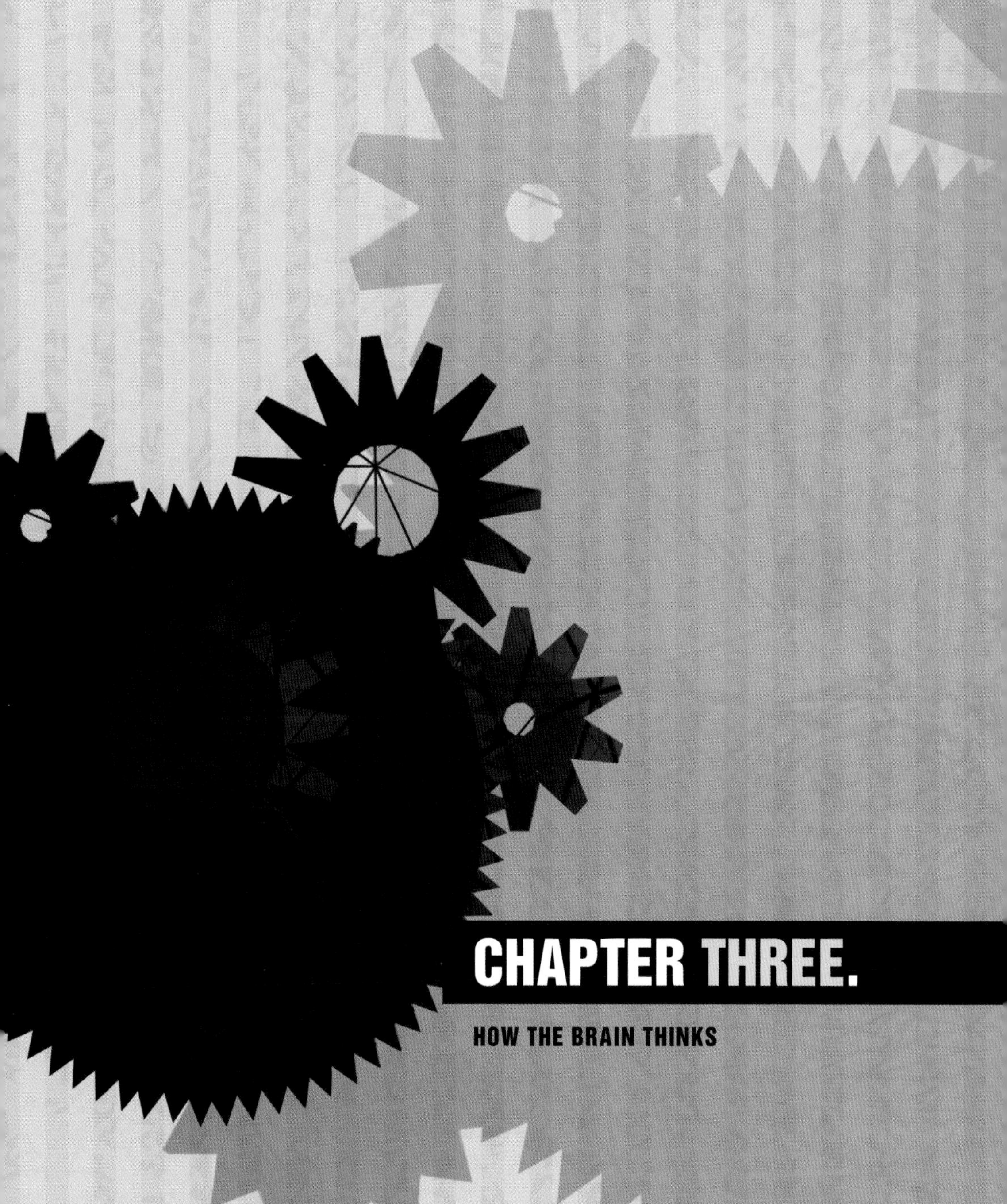

CHAPTER THREE.

HOW THE BRAIN THINKS

THREE.

HOW THE BRAIN THINKS

How to use the left and right sides of the brain for sporting excellence

THE LEFT SIDE OF THE BRAIN

The brain goes into autopilot and will use a preferred side when learning new skills.

It is important to remember that memory is stored in all parts of the brain.

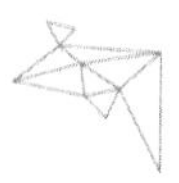

"I am the greatest; I said that even before I knew I was." Muhammad Ali

THIS IS WHAT HAPPENS IN THE LEFT SIDE OF THE BRAIN:

Analytical thinking pre and post-race—perhaps you think about if you had taken more or less calories per hour and how that could have impacted you going faster or slower. It also compares your splits to see how good your pace was throughout the run.

You set targets to achieve on the race day. How close were you and, if you weren't, why not? Was the course accurate and how good was the weather?

Congratulate yourself on your performance.

Work out your list of priorities for your next triathlon. Where can you improve? How good were you at sighting in the swim, how smooth were your transitions, and were you relaxed and quick? How quickly did you get into a cycling rhythm after swimming? Were you able to find your running legs after the biking within a few minutes? Did you hold a good pace for each discipline and, if not, why not?

The left side of the brain also helps analyze long-term goals, like how fast can I eventually get next month or next season or ever? This side of the brain is also used to work out your bank account balance.

THE RIGHT SIDE OF THE BRAIN

THIS IS WHAT HAPPENS IN THE RIGHT SIDE OF THE BRAIN:

The right side (hemisphere) of the brain is more sensitive to the emotional fears of language. It is used when driving.

STATES OF MIND

COMPARISON BETWEEN THE MIND AND A COMPUTER:

The conscious mind is like a keyboard and monitor. It is responsible for our awareness while we are awake. Here we process mental thoughts and talk rationally. Our memories are stored in our consciousness so that they can be retrieved and used. Sigmund Freud referred to this as our preconscious.

The subconscious mind is like a data processor that is active and has information that is quickly available. It is also referred to as the preconscious mind that operates below our normal consciousness. We retrieve ordinary memory information from our consciousness when it is required.

The unconscious mind is like the hard drive of your computer and its long-term storage space.

It is interchangeable with the subconscious mind and works outside the conscious mind. Here we have a reservoir of feelings, desires, thoughts and urges. This is where unpleasant thoughts are stored, including anxiety, conflict, pain, and bad experiences. With strong, positive, mental imagery these unpleasant thoughts can influence our lives, and they affect the way we react and make decisions.

Sigmund Freud, the famous Austrian psychoanalyst, believed that behavior and personality originated from different levels of awareness.

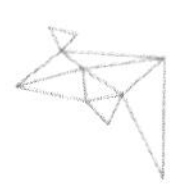

"Either you run the day or the day runs you." Jim Rohn

SCIENCE INSIDE THE BRAIN

Most parts of our anatomy are made up of two halves.

The brain is interconnected with a very high-speed network. Both sides process the same amount of input but use the information in a different way.

The left side of the brain controls the right side of the body, and the right side of the brain controls the left side. Therefore, the sensory data from your left eye is processed on the right side of the body.

For example, the right eye and the right hand can identify a phone, but the left side of the brain that processes this information could not explain what it is used for. The left eye and left hand sends signals to the right side of the brain and knows how to use it but will not be able to explain what it was.

Understanding the basic principles of the brain helps one see that the left side processes verbal information and non-verbal information is processed in the right side of the brain. The most important factor is to know that both sides complement each other.

Most people never reach their maximum potential because of trying to "please" both sides of the brain. The best option can either be to use the left side for tasks with less skill or using logic, or the right side using creativity or imagination. We also use our age, past experiences, education and beliefs to make decisions. Having saved positive mental imagery for the future can help you in the future.

Make sure your decision does not use the "tip of the iceberg" analogy. Don't always make decisions on what you see rather than what you know. The iceberg comparison = small, white part visible and large, dark part hidden beneath the surface.

The conscious mind is responsible for being aware while awake. The analytical part of the brain puts everything into order, so if you struggle with this part during mental imagery, first make a list in chronological order. The conscious mind will be concerned about cause and effect.

TRIATHLON EXAMPLE USING ANALYTICAL THINKING

What if I see myself in the swim with faster swimmers—will I be able to get a draft and be pulled along? What if I can't keep up? Will I get repeatedly swum over? If you practice this in training with a buddy who can swim faster, you can experience what it is like and see if you can recover after the initial surge behind faster swimmers before trying it for the first time in a triathlon. By doing this, you will have the facts to make the correct decision.

You think "I have not done enough training"

This is your logical solution to the problem. Rather than worry that you have not done much training for your triathlon and rather than compare yourself with someone else who has done more, this type of thinking will build doubt in your mind. Find out who was able to complete the triathlon on less training than you have done.

Most people have a preference for using one side of the brain more than the other side. It is highly unlikely that we are right- or left-brain dominant, but people are more comfortable with learning in a particular way, either audibly or visually. You may have a more dominant side of the body, say with the left side, with a dominant eye or foot, or have more dexterity on one side.

Personality comes from how the two sides interact or clash, or which side takes control.

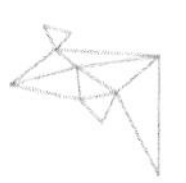

> **"The will to win, the desire to succeed, the urge to reach your full potential, these are the keys that will unlock the door to personal excellence."** Confucius

It is not the size of the brain that matters but how you process the information and then use it.

Neanderthals had a brain of 1500 cc, which was larger than today's humans, but were never able to use it to the best of its capacity. Our ancestors had a brain size of 1200 cc whereas modern day man's size is 1400 cc, yet geniuses' brains have varied in size from 1000 cc to 2000 cc. One quarter of our daily requirements is used for energy for the brain.

Facial expressions are the earliest form of our ancestor's communication, and after we are born, it's used as expression. To improve your success rate in a competition, add expressions when saving mental preparation imagery. Then when you are pushing to the finish with a smile, you will be reinforcing that all is well and feel it is ok to continue and not slow down. Many of the best sporting triathlon greats ran to the finishing line first with a smile.

These triathletes always had a smile while racing:

- Natasha Badman was Ironman® world triathlon champion in 1998, 2000, 2001, 2002, 2004 and 2005
- Chrissie Wellington was Ironman® world triathlon champion in 2007, 2008, 2009 and 2011
- Simon Whitfield won gold at the inaugural Olympics in Sydney in 2000
- Greg Welch won at the Olympics in 1990 and was Ironman® world triathlon champion in 1994
- Siri Lindley was the World Olympic distance champion in 2001
- More recently, Pete Jacobs was Ironman® world triathlon champion in 2012

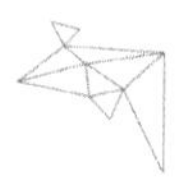

"If you can dream it, you can do it." Walt Disney

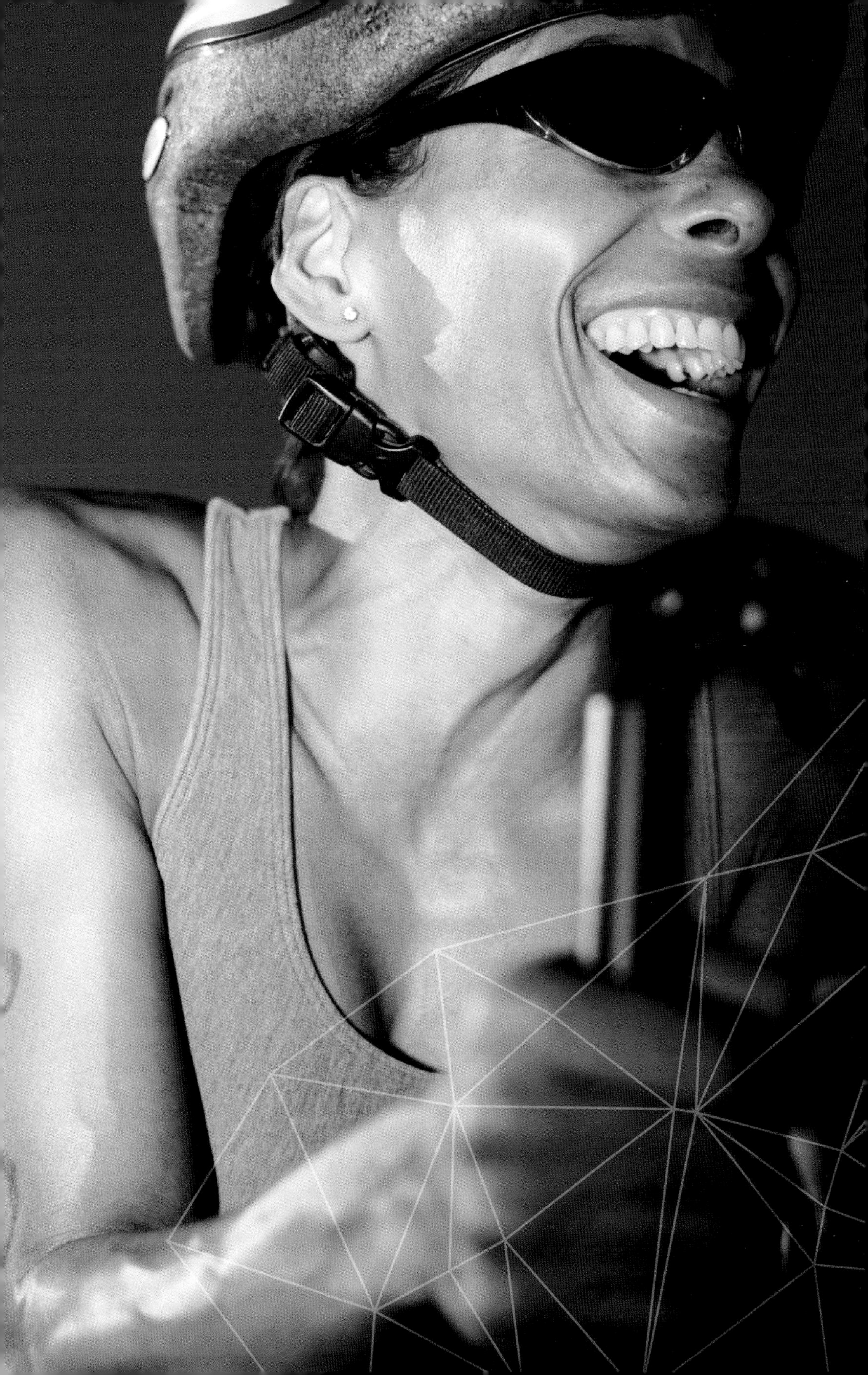

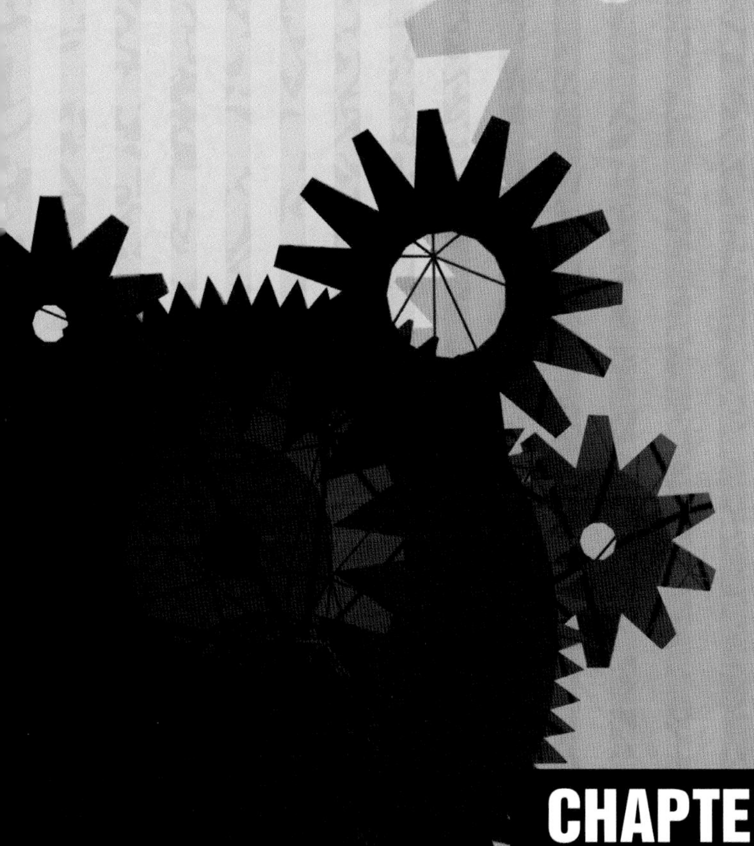

CHAPTER FOUR.

EFFECTIVE COPING STRATEGIES

FOUR.
EFFECTIVE COPING STRATEGIES

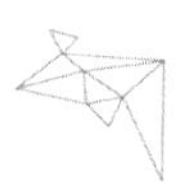

"No one can make you feel inferior without your consent."
Eleanor Roosevelt

"It's all in the Mind"

When a computer gets too much conflicting information, it crashes. When the human mind has too much information, it cannot make the correct decisions. Use the experience and information you have learned and process this to go into autopilot when you need to make a decision. Emotions often cause you to make the wrong decisions.

Concentration is a vital aspect of sporting excellence. You first need to establish what causes you to lose your concentration.

Have a ritual warm-up linking linked with concentration. Use sunglasses to prevent eye contact with others or use headphones can be switched on/off to prevent fellow competitors from speaking to you.

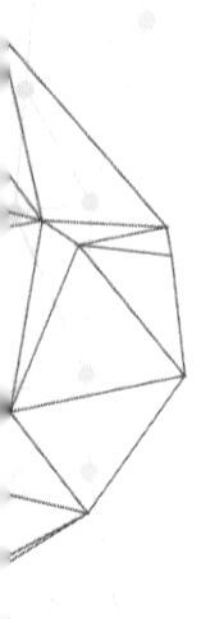

CONCENTRATION EXERCISE:

1. Breathing–Sit in an upright supportive chair with both arms and feet uncrossed. Close your eyes and take in deep breaths. Then exhale slowly, really focusing on your chest expanding and relaxing.
2. Now think about your breathing and concentrate on any aspect of your triathlon. Using a picture can really make a difference. Think about every little detail for at least 2 minutes. This can be a picture of you competing.

3. Now close your eyes and think of the image. Then think about competing in the triathlon.
4. To be more triathlon specific, try to close your eyes. Sit still for at least 5 minutes.

COMPETITION INTENSITIES

There are three basic intensities: under-intensity, race pace intensity and over-intensity.

Under-intensity will never harm your race performance as it allows you to hydrate, digest calories, and relax tight muscles. As soon as you realize you are in the under-intensity range then it is time to build back into race pace intensity, unless of course you cannot be caught from behind.

Race pace intensity is the pace you can maintain for the duration of the triathlon without slowing down. Most triathletes train much harder than this pace, falsely believing that fast training will help them go faster during competition. In reality, it's not the lack of speed that slows you down; it's the slowing down at the end. If you don't believe me then just look at 95% of the top 50 run splits in any triathlon. The one who slows down least or is the last one to slow down is usually the winner.

Over-intensity occurs when you are passing a competitor, trying to stay ahead or making a final push, and this should be avoided for the majority of the competition. Be careful when trying too hard because if you back off, you could slow down too much. Spending just 4 minutes too hard at the swim start will affect the later part of your triathlon and often result in a disappointing performance.

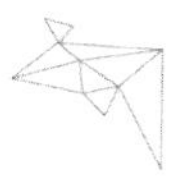

"An error is caused by learning, a mistake is letting that error happen again." Mark Kleanthous

MENTAL REHEARSAL TECHNIQUES

Do you know why an even heart rate and an even pacing is better than going off fast and then slowing down?

If you over-extend yourself during a triathlon, you simply have to slow down. Once this happens, you reduce the blood flow to the working muscles, which contain oxygen and adrenaline necessary for agility, strength and stamina. Then you will experience a further decline in performance, which can then have a negative impact on your motivation.

Following these easy-to-follow techniques will help you be sufficiently psyched and ready to race.

INTENSE BREATHING

Deep breathing can reduce the intensity of a hard workout and also help with getting back to a higher intensity. If your performance declines, take a few deep breaths to help increase the intensity again.

ENTHUSIASTIC SELF-TALK

Keep your mind believing and your body will follow. Let your mind give up and almost straightaway your body also gives up. Disappointing thoughts send body language signals to ease back, slow down or give up. A focused mind can still be motivated. Counteract these thoughts like a boxer would at the height of a fight with high-energy thoughts.

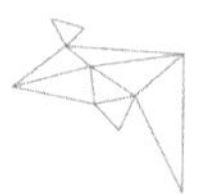

"Twenty years from now you will be more disappointed by the things you didn't do that by the ones you did do." Mark Twain

INCREASE THE INTENSITY THROUGH CHANGE

In training, establish how to increase the intensity with movement. If you are a strength athlete, do you need to have a faster arm turnover for swimming? If you are an endurance athlete with lots of slow-twitch muscles, do you need to use your strength more for a short period of time? This can get you race ready or back into your selected pace, so you may only need to do this different physical action for 30 seconds. Find out what works best for you.

Mentality mindset with tunnel vision focus allows the triathlete to stick to the task. Be sure to realize when it would be wiser to complete the workout indoors rather than complete the planned schedule, for instance when it is icy outside or there is a high probability of injury.

Nervousness is normal and can be channeled to help performance. Overcome obstacles and difficult situations during preparation in training and on race day.

Be passionate about triathlon and being a triathlete each and every day. Passion is needed to keep training. Then keep going on race day irrespective of ability, age, and time available to train ability or talent.

Strive for the best possible race result or performance that you could possibly achieve, especially when situations like the weather get in the way.

Look for the positive in a negative.

By using this book, you can develop the mindset of a well-disciplined and successful triathlete.

Toughing it out means to keep going. Rather than thinking about pushing to the end, break up the finish into small steps, one at a time. Concentrate on the here and now.

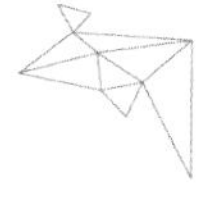

"The greatest danger for most of us is not that we aim to high and we miss it, but we aim to low and reach it." Michelangelo

VISUALIZATION

Training makes you leaner or bigger, stronger or faster or a combination. You can see the external results, but few triathletes including some of the best in the world practice daily mental training routine.

Mental rehearsal technique training

This is how a triathlete should first start mental visualization training.

You will need a quiet place–turn off your mobile phone, radio, television, etc.

You will need a sports drink.

Record what images you used for each of the senses.

Sit as comfortably as possible, then close your eyes.

Take at least 30 seconds to relax, taking deep breaths.

Then start to imagine.

VISUAL (SEEING) IMAGES IN THE MIND

Imagine a relaxing setting. It is no good to imagine lying on a hot beach if you find this uncomfortable or if you are prone to sunburn, or if you struggle to lie still for 5 minutes. Instead, think of a relaxing situation.

Try and imagine each sense one after the other.

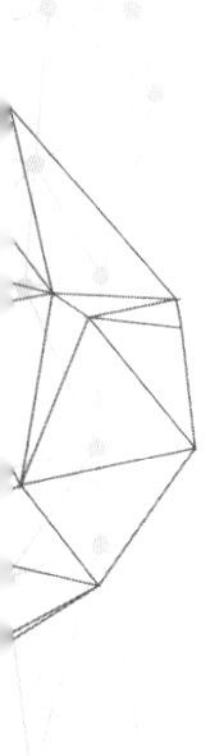

SENSE OF SMELL (OLFACTORY)

Try to imagine the smell of a great tasting food you enjoy.

SENSE OF SOUND (HEARING)

Imagine the sound of people chatting at a near-by table in a restaurant.

SENSE OF FEELING (KINESTHETIC)

Relax all your muscles.

SENSE OF TASTE (GUSTATORY)

Try and think about the taste sensations of your favorite food–freshly baked bread or coffee–then progress to race morning breakfast race nutrition and hydrating flavored drinks.

Before you stop visualizing, think of which sense you found the easiest to recall and hold onto.

Easier senses will still need to be worked on but these will be the ones you try and start mental rehearsal with before incorporating the more difficult senses.

Before finishing, the mental training should be more triathlon sport specific:

Image thought–A famous triathlete that you admire. Notice how smooth they look when they swim, bike and run, then imagine yourself following them.

Smell sensation–Progress to imagining the smell of your swim cap or neoprene wetsuit, or a new piece of equipment or clothing.

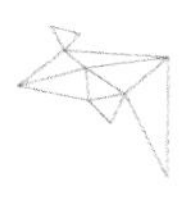

"A mind is like a parachute. It doesn't work if it isn't open."
Frank Zappa

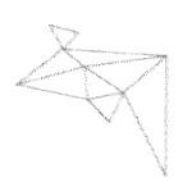

"Don't go through life, grow through life." Eric Butterworth

VISUAL (SEEING) IMAGES IN THE MIND

Imagine a relaxing setting. This could be having a massage or warm bath or simply lying still reading a good book.

Sound sensations–The noise at the start of the triathlon, the sound of arms and legs thrashing in the open water.

Feeling sensation—Recall feelings of yourself getting into the water to swim, the air on your face as you cycle along, and the sweat pouring down your face as you run.

Taste sensations—While your eyes are closed, sip a sports drink.

How do these sport specific sensations affect you?

Consider temperature sensations, the air then water temperature; the air passing by you on the bike.

The above was a dress rehearsal for visualizing more using triathlon details.

SPORT SPECIFIC MENTAL PERFORMANCE PRACTICE

You need a quiet place, usually at home on your own away from outside distractions. It can involve thinking about a new skill like improved stroke technique, cycling action, or running light on your feet.

You can use mental imagery when the weather or other circumstances like being injured or ill make it impossible to train.

It is even more important to complete mental visualization when you cannot train because you need to keep the nervous system focused on the skills of your sport. You are far more likely to resume quicker and potentially better than where you stopped by mentally rehearsing.

Now you are ready.

Take a moment to consider what you need to focus on. Try to avoid fast-forwarding through a triathlon because it is unlikely to benefit you as much as taking your time.

Imagine the setting at the beginning of the triathlon; you have already prepared your transition.

You now see the lake and then you see yourself walking (relaxed) into your image. You look at the buoys, place the swim goggles on your face and then enter to waist-deep in the water. Double check the route you are about to take.

Visualize yourself feeling warm wearing the correct type of goggles (tinted for a bright day, clear for an overcast day).

Try to feel the weather conditions you expect race morning.

Take some deep breaths, look at your stopwatch and press it to start. Swim at a good pace, not too hard so you don't end up exhausted. Imagine the sounds you may hear under your swim cap.

Feel the water as your hand enters the water, catching and pulling through the water.

During your mental imagery, you observe and listen to other swimmers around you making their own little noises.

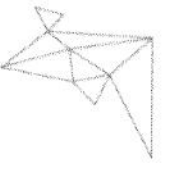

"Worrying is like a rocking chair. It gives you something to do but it doesn't get you anywhere." Van Wilder

CHAPTER FIVE.

HOW TO CHANGE YOUR ATTITUDE

FIVE.

HOW TO CHANGE YOUR ATTITUDE

PSYCH-UP TECHNIQUES FOR TRIATHLETES

Did you know that a constant heart rate with even pacing is better than going off fast and then slowing down?

If you over-extend yourself during a triathlon, you simply have to slow down. If you don't slow down, you reduce the blood flow to the working muscles, which contain the oxygen and adrenaline necessary for agility, strength and stamina. Then you will experience a further decline in performance, which can then have a negative impact on your motivation.

By following these easy techniques, you will be sufficiently psyched and ready to race.

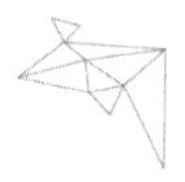

"The best way to predict the future is to invent it." Alan Kay

KEY WORDS TO KEEP ON TRACK

Focus on key words to lower the intensity—try telling yourself to "stay calm" or "it's better if I hold back a little." You can also use key words with confidence to increase the pace like "stay strong" or "those around me are struggling."

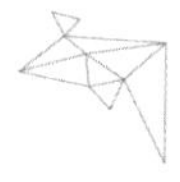

"It's your thinking that decides whether you're going to succeed or fail." Henry Ford

FAKING BODY LANGUAGE

Fake by making yourself look strong and composed and combine this with enthusiastic self-talk. This results in signals that will be sent around the body saying that all is well and then you will carry on with greater passion.

QUIET TIME—USEFUL TIPS AND TECHNIQUES

- Quiet moment while brushing your teeth; or go to bed 10 minutes early and before you fall asleep.
- I am the captain of my ship and master of my fate.
- Stay away from negative people.
- During quiet moments, repeat your mantra.

How to clear the mind of stress and clutter:

Like anything, it takes practice so do not give up if you can't clear the mind after 15 seconds of your first-ever attempt.

Work for 90 minutes, take a break, then continue–known as "pulsing". Some athletes in endurance events concentrate for a set period of 40-90 minutes, then when safe to do so, they clear the mind of thoughts for 60 seconds and then get back to 100% concentration.

Busy lives can be fulfilling but they can cause mental overload, stress and anxiety that transfer to family work and triathlons. Anxiety from life that is totally unrelated to sport can manifest itself in even the slightest of worries you may have had for open water swimming or descending down a hill.

- Sync your breath with movement.
- Gently walk, connect with nature, stop and sit outside and watch birds flying, or even better watch a river running, watch ripples on a lake or stare out into the ocean.
- Sing in the shower, car, in a choir or out on your own while training.

- Make a favorite meal, try nothing new, and don't fret or worry about making it perfect because this will just add stress.
- Do something you love. Listen to relaxing music, practice yoga, write a poem, read a favorite part of a book, or just focus on one thing and avoid wild or distracting thoughts.
- Exercise with ease, as the body moving can be very therapeutic.
- Buy flowers and smell them at any opportunity then close your eyes for 10 seconds while smelling them again.
- Call a friend you have not spoken to in a while.
- Write down your dreams and aspirations and once you have made your list, close your mind and relax for a while and think of these thoughts.
- Have a cuddle because it will release hormones to make you feel good.
- Watch a comedian or your favorite film of fun things on YouTube.
- Find a quiet space to be alone and enjoy your own time and your own company.
- Have a warm relaxing bath. Add oils and mineral salts and unwind. Just feel the warmth on your body and switch off your busy mind.

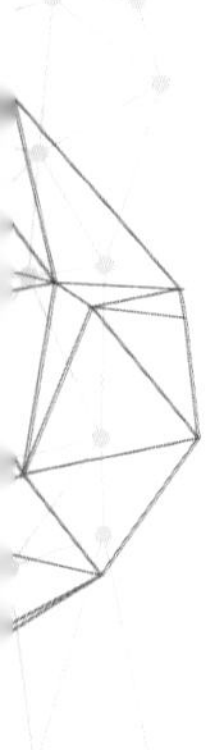

Get into the zone, and prepare yourself every day. Our minds are far more active than our bodies.

It does not have to take up extra time. Mental imagery can be done anywhere, anytime, or any place. Use your senses to get more into the experience.

Think about the triathlon on the toilet seat and how you will feel race morning when on the toilet.

While having a cold shower, visualize a cold swim or it being cooler than expected.

When in a hot sauna, think about it being a hot race day. When you get hungry, think about being low on energy on race day and how nutrition can pick you up.

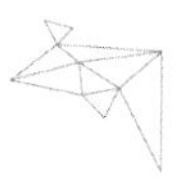

> "The difference between a successful person and others is not a lack of strength, not a lack of knowledge, but rather a lack of will."
> Vince Lombardi

PHYSICAL REHEARSAL TECHNIQUES

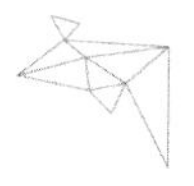

> "The successful warrior is the average man, with laser like focus."
> Bruce Lee

BREATHING

Breathing is probably the most under-appreciated of all the human activities; we breathe an average of 20,000 times a day. Constriction in breathing can lead to subpar mental performance, fatigue, mild depression, poor athletic performance, and even heart attacks.

Your brain uses four times more oxygen than any other part of the body. The brain is the first part of the body to be affected from shallow or restricted breathing.

Stress can impact our breathing. When we are under stress, we tend to hold our breath. Lifting heavy weights, bench-pressing, sit-ups, pull-ups, dips, and pull-downs can tighten the shoulder muscles, which also restricts our breathing.

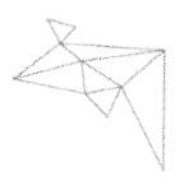

> "I find the harder I work, the more luck I seem to have."
> Thomas Jefferson

CHAPTER SIX.

STRESS FACTORS AND HOW TO USE THEM TO YOUR ADVANTAGE

SIX.

STRESS FACTORS AND HOW TO USE THEM TO YOUR ADVANTAGE

6.1 AGE

The older you are, the more you should use mental imagery to enhance sporting performance. Totally eliminate any errors. Athletes who perform better than they did a decade before do so due to using mental imagery.

A body scan is even more important once we reach our mid-30s. Warm up, then stretch to feel for signs of tightness. On rest days or the day after a recovery day, we often notice any issues that were hidden during training days.

Take corrective measures if you have a slight ache, like having a massage, getting treatment, icing an area, or not running. Instead, complete a drill swim set.

As your body ages, it becomes less flexible. Strength and speed are reduced but experience increases.

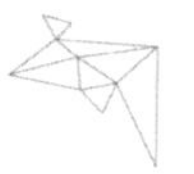

"Age is an issue of mind over matter. If you don't mind, it does not matter." Mark Twain

There are also more frequent injuries and strains, with recovery time taking much longer. Consider this when preparing your training plan.

6.2 BACKGROUND

In the 19th century, sports were considered mainly as a leisure pursuit. The working class athletes back then did not have leisure time, and only the wealthy could take time off from work to take part in sports. If the working class did participate, they did it for money because they lost wages while not working.

Social class can affect the mindset of a triathlete and their will to succeed. People from every social background have probably competed in triathlons during the last 35 years of the sport's existence.

Triathlon can be an expensive sport with all the equipment and cost of travelling, entry fees, etc., so it may exclude those with little disposable income.

To excel in sport you need nature and nurture. Nature is having the best genetics passed to you by your parents. Nurture is the right environment, support and guidance from your parents and coaches.

The limiting factor for endurance athletes is cardiac capacity. The heart's ability to deliver enough oxygen via the blood stream to the skeletal muscles is important, and is dependent on your genetics.

Being successful in sport can depend on the sports your parents played. Most single discipline sports clubs now have a small percentage of triathletes trying to improve their individual disciplines.

Today, most people have more leisure time and can compete every weekend if they want to. The term "Weekend Warrior" is for people who compete at the weekend. Some are serious and train meticulously while others do the minimum to get by at the weekend competitions.

In triathlon like the marathon, you can be in an amateur age group and compete in the same event as full-time professionals. The best triathletes have come from a swimming background and then progressed to running and cycling. Few world-class single sport athletes (swimmers, cyclists, rowers, and runners) have been successful in switching and being competitive at triathlon in a few months as there is much to teach the body and the mind.

Motivation and nutrition also help in sporting performance.

Like any sport, triathlon can have a positive or negative impact on family life.

Some people have met because of triathlon and found a happy balance between competing and sharing precious time together while others have blamed their divorces on triathlon.

To be successful, you will need to train the mind and the body for many years to reach peak performance, so without motivation you are unlikely to succeed. Sir David Brailsford has been responsible for British cycling success by choosing athletes who are highly motivated.

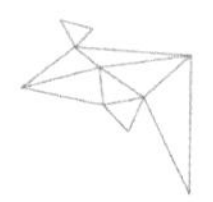

"A pessimist sees the difficulty in every opportunity; an optimist sees the opportunity in every difficulty." Sir Winston Churchill

6.3 GENDER

The differences between males and females are due mainly to physiology. On average, men are stronger due to their body composition, while their heart and lungs are generally larger.

A typical man can have half as much fat and around twice as much muscle as a woman of similar size. Men can also run faster than women due to having a larger heart and lungs.

With a man taking more breaths per minute than a woman, he has the advantage in most endurance events.

Surprisingly, fewer women take part in sport than men. Unlike men, women often need to juggle family life, especially with the children, with their sporting pursuits.

This becomes difficult because they need to train for many hours in order to become psychologically fit and competitive. This is much easier to achieve for men.

Sport for women comes with various risks, such as the fact that they are often subject to the control and influence of male teachers and coaches. This can lead to a risk of harassment.

For women in sport there are also the problems of menstruation, menopause, osteoporosis, and even eating disorders that can seriously affect concentration and performance.

There is a difference in strength between women and men primarily due to the anabolic effect of testosterone in men's muscular system. It's therefore very important for the woman to gain muscular strength.

Sport-related injuries are higher in women regarding the overuse of muscles and joints.

Despite all of the above concerns, some of the best female endurance triathletes and athletes regularly finish in the top 2% overall and often beat many professional male triathletes.

6.4 SPORTING EXPERIENCE

The difference between an error and a mistake is an error is hindsight—looking back and learning from a poor decision; a mistake is ignoring what you experienced before or doing what you were told not to do.

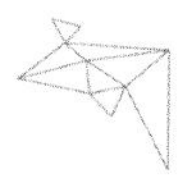

> **"A man who views the world the same at fifty as he did at twenty has wasted thirty years of his life."** Muhammad Ali

Although stress is a negative factor to achieving success because it can lead to burnout, it can also be used positively. Sports people can use the fight-or-flight technique in order to win an event.

One needs to have balance and have enough pressure to focus on goals, but not too much because it could disrupt overall performance.

Use your past sporting experiences by mentally rehearsing what you have learned in the past to improve.

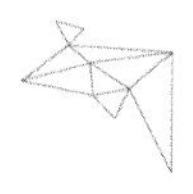

> **"It is not whether you get knocked down, it's whether you get up."** Vince Lombard

6.5 LIFESTYLE

Having a laugh or a giggle reduces stress chemicals that strengthen the immune system.

Make a checklist of things to do. For some people, this may initially increase your stress levels, but once you see what you have to do and prioritize it all and then tick off things you have done, stress levels soon drop.

Take some quiet time. Even 5 minutes lying in the bath and switching off all your thoughts can work wonders. But don't relax so much that you fall asleep!

Listening to relaxing music before you go to sleep can also improve the quality of your sleep.

6.6 NUTRITION

There are many ways to boost your mood, which helps with reducing stress. For example, foods we eat affect our emotions. Dairy products are a good source of the amino acid tryptophan, which is needed by the body to make mood-boosting serotonin. Omega 3 fatty acids obtained from beef, flax seeds, salmon, sardines, scallops, shrimp, soybeans and walnuts can reduce fatigue, which boosts serotonin levels.

Feel-good factor foods contain tryptophan. Tryptophan is one of the ten essential amino acids that the body requires to synthesize proteins.

Tryptophan is vital for relaxation, restfulness and sleep because it is necessary for the creation of serotonin that is vital to regulate appetite, sleep patterns and mood.

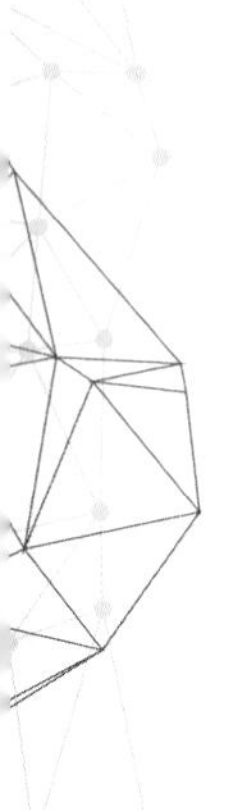

Foods that contain tryptophan are listed below:

- Dairy products
- Legumes
- Nuts
- Red meat
- Seeds

- Shellfish
- Chicken
- Soybeans
- Soy products
- Turkey
- Tuna
- Lamb
- Salmon
- Halibut
- Shrimp
- Cod and sardines
- Tofu
- Spinach
- Asparagus
- Dried peas
- Kidney beans
- Pumpkin seeds
- Lentils
- Cow's milk (grass fed)
- Eggs (free range)

A dietary deficiency of tryptophan may lead to low levels of serotonin. Low serotonin levels are associated with depression, anxiety, irritability, impatience, impulsiveness, an inability to concentrate, weight gain, overeating, carbohydrate cravings, poor dream recall, and insomnia.

The following lifestyle factors—excess alcohol, cigarette smoking, high sugar intake, and large amounts of protein—reduce the effectiveness of converting tryptophan into serotonin.

Feel-good factor foods include:

- Bananas can help keep you from "going bananas" because they contain tryptophan plus B6. The banana is rich in mood-boosting carbohydrates.

- Brazil nuts contain selenium—people with anxiety, depression or those always feeling tired have low levels of selenium. These nuts can be eaten with a breakfast or snack and even chopped into a salad.
- Dark chocolate causes a release of endorphins that boosts serotonin levels. Some studies have found that eating chocolate for two weeks lowers stress hormones being released and then anxiety levels drop. Dark chocolate is better than milk chocolate but make sure it contains 70% cocoa solids, which are rich in antioxidants.
- Lentils are a complex carbohydrate, and they help increase serotonin to make you calmer, happier and less anxious. They contain folic acid, which can reduce depression. They are also rich in iron, which helps you feel less tired.
- Oats have a low glycemic index that avoids energy highs and lows and helps maintain a constant blood sugar level. Selenium contained in oats helps regulate the thyroid gland.
- Protein (chicken eggs and fish) should be eaten twice a day. Aim for two smaller portions rather than one large portion once a day.
- Sardines contain Omega 3, so if you are susceptible to low mood swings or depression, make sure you get enough oily fish. Enough Omega 3 helps with the brain working more efficiently.
- Spinach contains vitamin B, so if you are deficient, you are more likely to suffer from depression. Vitamin B helps serotonin production.
- Herbal tea (chamomile), known as a cup of calm, will help you relax by staving off depression. Licorice manufacturers claim it is a powerful anti-depressant and can even help with mouth ulcers.
- Yogurt contains vitamin D, which is also obtained from

sunlight via our skin. It is important to take it in times of stress and to prevent anxiety. This is especially true during the winter when there is less daylight and you may spend more time indoors.

- Water is needed every day to keep us hydrated and help with concentration.
- Optimists eat more carotenoids and pessimists tend to eat less. By increasing carotenoids in their diet, pessimists can increase their feel-good factors and improve their positive outlook on life, training and competing. The triathlete will really benefit from focusing on foods that help with mood and reduction of stress.
- Foods rich in carotenoids include carrots, fruits, grapefruit, pink pumpkins, sweet potatoes, vegetables and watermelons.

ANTIOXIDANTS

Antioxidants are a substance that prevents damage or destruction by oxidation. Oxygen is a vitally important element of our existence, however when oxygen is used, free radicals are released and oxidation occurs, which can be damaging to the human body. This causes damage to tissues, memory and moods, hardening of the arteries and joints stiffening.

The older the triathlete, the more oxidation occurs in the human body. This happens to everything from butter turning rancid to fruits turning brown and metals rusting.

Antioxidants for body maintenance are good, and free radicals are bad. The more you can protect your cells, the more you can reduce aging and help with recovery.

Exposure to environmental toxins in the air we breathe, water we drink, and certain foods that we eat, increases free radical damage. The human body has an amazing ability to handle free radicals, but once there is too much, it can cause premature aging and disease.

Free radicals that can cause damage are found in the following:

- Alcohol
- Chemicals (household, fuel fumes)
- Chemotherapy (X-rays, TV and computer monitors)
- Cigarette smoke
- Coffee
- Colorings
- Drugs
- Fizzy drinks
- Hydrogenated and saturated fats
- Junk foods (margarines and oils)
- Medications
- Processed foods
- Refined foods (canned, frozen and white flour)
- Tap water
- Tea
- Temperature (too cold or hot)

NATURAL ANTIOXIDANTS

They minimize the effects of free radical damage and are found in plant foods. Without enough natural antioxidants, free radical damage can make you more susceptible to disease.

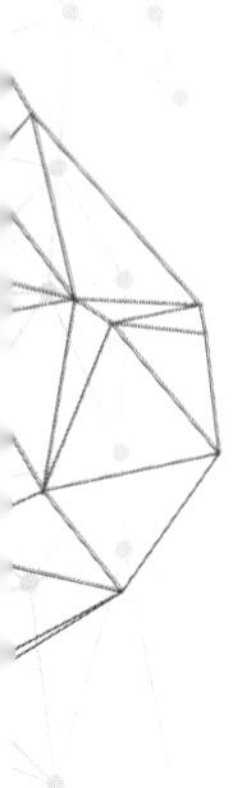

Foods Rich in Antioxidants

- Fresh fruits (not processed with skin)
- Fresh vegetables (not processed with skin)
- Eggs (free range)
- Herbs
- Meats (free range)
- Oils (cold press, canola, flax and olive oil)
- Nuts (raw)

- Organic varieties are generally higher in antioxidants:
- Raw foods
- Seaweeds
- Sprouts
- Unrefined foods
- Vegetables
- Whole foods (unprocessed) like fresh fruit, vegetables and nuts

Foods that are rich in vitamin B, C, and E can reduce free radical damage. They include the following:

- Avocado
- Aloe vera (cold press only)
- Apricots
- Apples
- Beetroots
- Blackberries
- Blueberries
- Carrots
- Cherries
- Citrus fruits
- Cranberries
- Oranges
- Pears
- Strawberries
- Vegetables

ANXIETY AND FOOD

We have all felt anxiety during our lives, from that first kiss to the job interview. Our heart is racing and we can feel it pounding in our chest so we get stressed. There are ways to reduce stress, such as slowing things down, which helps us become calm and relaxed. Emotion-busting remedies include the following:

Anxiety attacks can be triggered by a drop in blood sugar, so a gel with water just before a triathlon or a snack during the day can reduce anxiety.

Chamomile can help to calm the brain. If taken for 8 weeks, this can reduce problems with ongoing anxiety problems.

Lavender aroma helps with a sense of calm and lavender pills reduce anxiety.

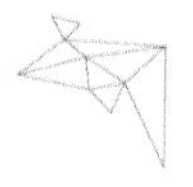

"You can't put a limit on anything. The more you dream, the farther you get." Michael Phelps

If you are trying to improve your mood, avoid foods like alcohol, caffeine, and sugar!

If you are craving salty foods like potato chips then you may have adrenal exhaustion from a 24/7 fast-paced life. Salt cravings are also linked to diabetes, high bloodpressure and other health issues.

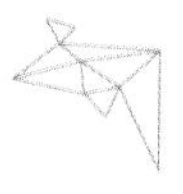

"Be miserable or motivate yourself. Whatever has to be done, it's always your choice." Wayne Dyer

6.7 SLEEP

Sleep can help a triathlete.

Brain cells shrink during sleep, which causes gaps to open between the neurons, and this allows fluid to wash between them and remove waste toxins. This cleanses the brain. Sleep is vital for recovery but is important for remembering and saving what we learned that day. Our brains have a limited amount of energy so sleeping is like turning our computer off and rebooting it when it slows down.

Restoration of brain functions while we sleep allows neurotoxins to be flushed away, and skills we have learned from the previous day are saved for the future.

Sleep can help cognitive skills bcause we sleep to remember. Everyone needs different amounts and this will vary depending on age, stress levels and training volumes.

Race week training is like a new open water swim environment—you improve the skill while sleeping. It is vital for staying awake and being alert the next day because it can help us learn. While we sleep, we enhance our memories.

Before I discuss this, let's look at the phases of sleep and what happens in each one:

SLEEP PHASES

Phase 1—In non-rapid eye movement (NREM) sleep, the brain gets slower and the brain neurons fire at a greater synchrony. If you wake up, you believe you have been awake and not fallen asleep. This is when we experience hypnotic jerks or involuntary twitches and movements.

Phase 2—This makes up the majority of our sleep. Dreaming is less common in this phase, and you can easily be woken.

Phase 3—This is short wave sleep (SWS) and NREM. This is our deepest stage of non-REM sleep. Electroencephalograms (EEG) measure electrical activity of the brain. These found high-amplitude and slow oscillations in electrical activity, meaning that the peaks and troughs were caused by the neurons acting in synchrony. During this phase, actylcholine (which keeps the brain awake) is twice the level when we are awake. This alters the connections between the neurons and allows new links, which helps with learning and remembering new skills.

RAPID EYE MOVEMENT (REM) SLEEP

The eyes are closed but there are darting movements under the closed eyelids. This is when we have emotional dreams. Unlike shortwave sleep, the brain is not synchronised, so activity is happening and appears to be in a haphazard way all over the brain. This brain activity continues when we are awake.

The better quality sleep we get, the better our memories improve, which can reinforce our mental imagery and the timing can make it even more beneficial.

So what does that all mean for a triathlete? You are likely to get more REM in the morning and more SWS in the afternoon or evening.

Planning the time for a power nap is vital to get the most specific benefit. Scientists believe that dreams are memories being played back, and most people improve skills when they have dreamt about them.

If practising mental imagery of your triathlon, especially if you can get emotional and passionate about the race, do this before a power nap in the morning.

Plan on studying the race details, looking at your training diary, detailing heart rate data or improving technique. Consider a power nap in the afternoon because this is a good time for the mind to store these memories while asleep.

6.8 HEALTH

BREATHING

When you race up to half an Ironman® event distance, your breathing needs to be controlled. During intense exercise, your breathing also needs to be controlled so avoid short choppy breathing, which results in not getting enough oxygen. Instead, deep breathe to get the most amount of oxygen into the lungs to be transported around the body. Even when exercising at a high intensity, you can become relaxed by deep breaths, so feeling calmer can help with overcoming negative thoughts caused by over sensitivity.

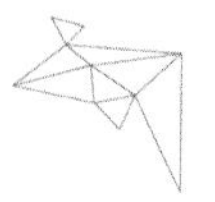

"If you want to conquer fear, don't sit home and think about it. Go out and get busy." Dale Carnegie

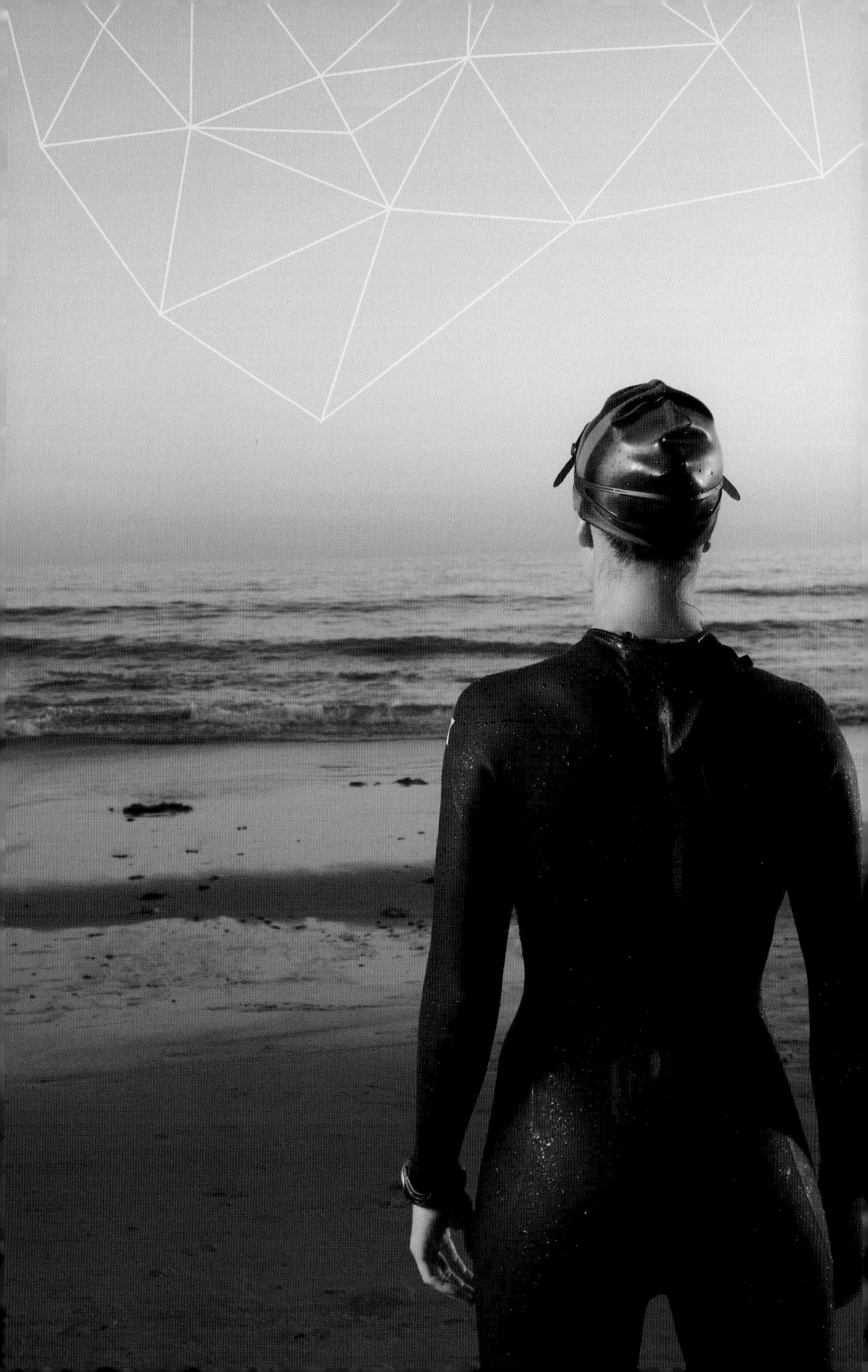

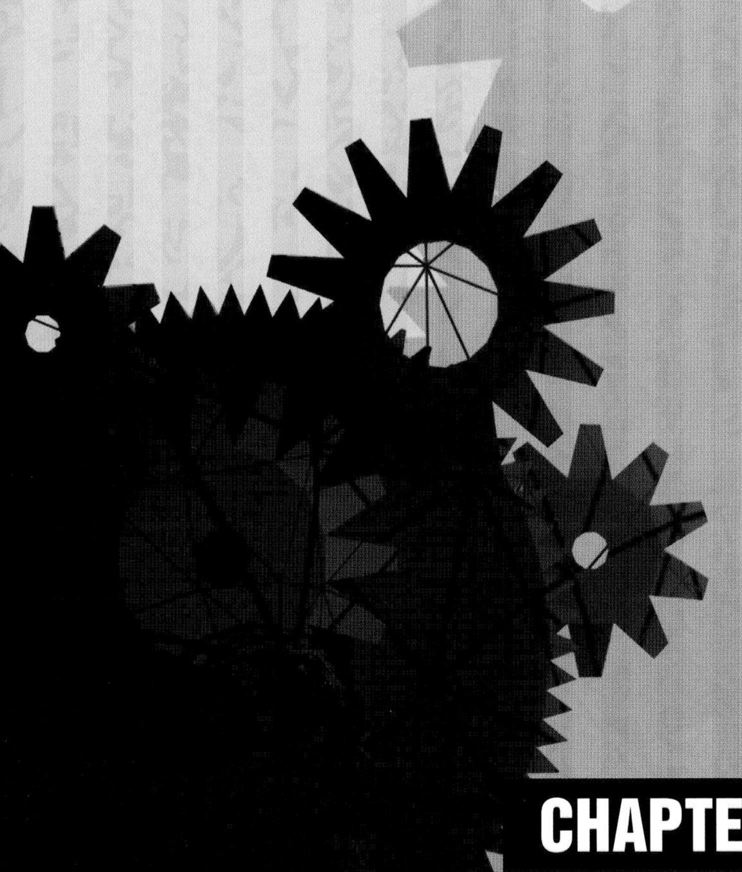

CHAPTER SEVEN.

DEMANDS OF THE EVENT

SEVEN.

DEMANDS OF THE EVENT

BEFORE A CHALLENGE

"What if I fail?"–Change this mindset to "no one who tries is a failure."

If I don't try then I will not fail–Change your mind to think you will be more dissappointed never knowing what you may have achieved.

A fixed mindset accepts failure.

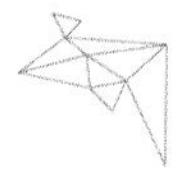

"The questions isn't who is going to let me, it's who is going to stop me." Ayn Rand

WHEN A PROBLEM OCCURS

Reorganize yourself, offer a choice and you can change your mind.

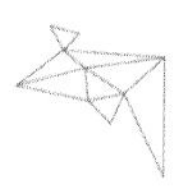

"Life is not about waiting for the storm to pass, it's about learning to dance in the rain." Vivian Greene

"I am worried about making mistakes."–Triathletes that learn from mistakes do not make excuses and thus improve in the future.

Growth mindset–All great triathletes have setbacks and successfully move on. They learn to take responsibilty.

"I am worried about making the wrong decision."–It's ok to blame yourself if you make an error, provided you learn to move on and don't make the same mistake.

HOW TO COMPETE AND BE MENTALLY STRONG IF YOU ARE UNDERTRAINED

I am not suggesting you should compete in a triathlon distance event if you have not been able to prepare properly.

This book is not about training the mind so that you can cut corners, it's about using the mind to achieve your genetic potential.

In reality, less than 10% of triathletes actually complete every session planned before a triathlon. So many factors can stop you from training. Many triathlon winners and champions talk about all the problems with injuries, illness, missed training workouts and accidents that they had before getting to the start line.

Always believe that there is someone worse off than you, who has had less time to train or is physically challenged.

TAPERING

In the final weeks before your triathlon, make sure you are consistent with your swimming, cycling and running, and complete back-to-back sessions rather than just one discipline.

Avoid sports nutrition during most workouts up to 10–15 days before your triathlon. Just drink plain water, and then practice your sports drinks and nutrition during the final 10-day taper period leading up to triathlon day.

Avoid going hungry after training. Make sure you focus on the golden time within 30 minutes of finishing—replenishing carbohydrates, then protein, then keep snacking.

TRIATHLON DAY

› Eat as much as you can digest that will not cause a stomach ache.

- Do not fret and get stressed because this will cause you to waste energy.
- Be meticulous with attention to detail and eat smaller snacks often.
- Hold back and make sure you get the right amount of calories and hydrate fastidiously.
- Make sure you replace your cycle drink bottle with care into the bike holder—you simply cannot afford to drop it and lose hydration.
- Don't miss an opportunity at any feed station—slow down and get what you need. Use your fitness and save your strength for when you are low on energy.
- Spin easy gears up hills and have a fast leg turnover during the run but avoid leg sapping and over striding.
- Pace yourself from the very first swim stroke and always hold back and have something in reserve.

CLOSED MINDSET

Don't blame others for your mistakes. Accept the blame for not thinking something through, resulting in what you now consider the wrong decision.

Negative thoughts hold you back—Talk back to the voice in your head and take back control.

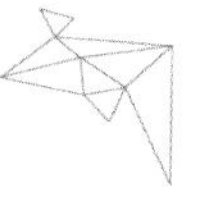

"Believe in yourself! Have faith in your abilities. Without a humble but reasonable confidence in your own powers you cannot be successful or happy." Norman Vincent Peale

UNFINISHED BUSINESS

All triathletes need to reflect after a triathlon. Straight after, a few days later, 7-10 days later; and then come to a conclusion. Avoid knee jerk decisions!

If you had a disappointing race then decide to compete again in two weeks before figuring out what went wrong then you are more than likely going to have a similarly poor performance.

Managing impulses will have a great influence on how successful you will be in the future.

Training has many health benefits but can also cause injuries.

Keeping focused or dealing with an injury physically and mentally is a major factor in future success. Many athletes fall by the wayside when they get injured, some ignore the warning signs and train through it while others don't do anything about it.

Remain positive and focused especially if you cannot train, avoid comfort foods that will make you put on weight, which will make the road back to fitness much longer.

When sport is an important part of your life and injury stops your training, the lack of endorphins, the loss of routine and the lack of identity will make you doubt your ability to become a successful triathlete. Being unable to train can cause a downward spiral of motivation because you are not achieving goals and either not performing as you would have hoped or not being able to compete in the triathlon.

This is where mental imagery can play a key role. Use your time wisely thinking about want you want to achieve once your injury has healed. It will improve your confidence, motivation and ability to fast track back once you are able to train again. Many athletes do not devote the time to mental practice so use this time while convalescing wisely.

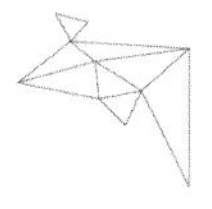

"If you can't get rid of the skeleton in your closet, you'd best teach it to dance." George Bernard Shaw

VOICES IN YOUR HEAD

Don't let the noise of other people's opinions drown out your inner voice. Process other people's words and follow the path led by your heart and intuition.

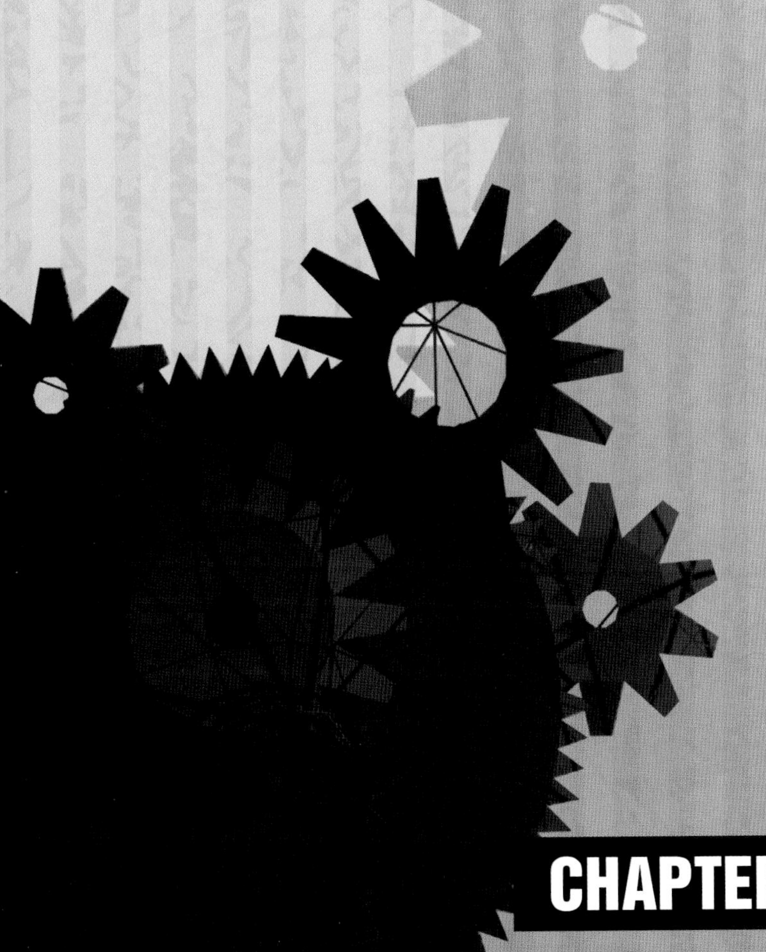

CHAPTER EIGHT.

OVERCOMING THE MIND

EIGHT.

OVERCOMING THE MIND

DEFEAT—COMPETITORS AND YOURSELF

Get energy from thinking the opposite. If you do not like being watched, learn to love being the center of attention.

We have two sides, a thinking and a performing part, and it is usually the thinking that inhibits us.

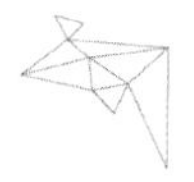

"Problems are not stop signs, they are guidelines."
Robert H. Schuller

LEARN TO OVERCOME GUIDELINES

If you have thought about what you want to do then you can do anything.

Mental imagery is dealing with attitude and how you want to shape the outcome.

When you actually compete in the triathlon, your mind already knows the procedure. Changing your attitude allows you more energy to focus on the whole task rather than one small part.

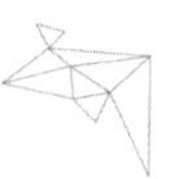

„Half this game is ninety percent mental." Yogi Berra

MUSIC FOR MOTIVATION

Few people are not motivated by music. Motivated triathletes can benefit from listening to certain soundtracks. Use music to psych yourself up or to keep to a rhythm or to pick yourself up or calm down. For me, music gives me excitement and energy, and if I am not training or racing, it makes me want to dance.

Your playlist could include a slow pace for a warm-up, fast for the main part or intervals and then gradually slow down

Only use music for motivation and remember many events do not allow you to listen to music, especially during a triathlon.

WAYS TO BEAT PRE-PERFORMANCE TRIATHLON NERVES

Almost everyone will experience stress at some time. It's the body's natural mechanism to help you get ready by releasing adrenaline to improve your focus.

If you worry too much, extra hormones are released that can cause you to become sweaty, get butterflies in the stomach, and not be able to think straight.

Psyching yourself up by telling yourself about how confident you can be combats stress hormones. You need to do this for many weeks or months before your competition then just feel your confidence grow.

Find a thought or image (such as a picture on your phone) that can help you relax and use this to calm and quiet down your mind.

Mimic what the experts use to mentally prepare.

Music helps but it must not be too upbeat to send your heartbeat racing. Some people need to be quiet with eyes closed, some need to chat, while others need to move a little. Establish what works best for you then keep practicing.

During race week when you may not train as much as you should but have a lot of things to do, make sure any spare time is not spent on the same image of events.

CRITICISM FROM WITHIN AND OTHERS

The pressure comes from within. Have a thick skin, and tunnel vision; ignore outside criticism! For some people, it is hard to swallow. Aim to use convert criticism in a constructive way.

When emotions become the dominant force it is difficult to make quality rational thoughts.

Praise yourself when no one else does.

Remember that (constructive) criticism is very important if you want to improve.

Our reaction or response is often based on our current state of emotion and how we perceive comments as negative or positive.

Few people achieved greatness without taking advice or ignoring constructive criticism.

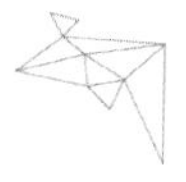

„It‘s not the size of the dog in the fight; it‘s the size of the fight in the dog.“ Mark Twain

LOSS OF CONFIDENCE

Uncertainty and no action will make you feel uncomfortable

Clear out negative thoughts and allow the rest of your mind to contribute positive thoughts.

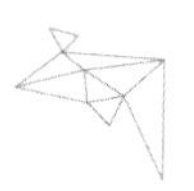

"I would rather attempt to do something great and fail than to attempt to do nothing and succeed." Robert H. Schuller

USE FEAR AS A POSITIVE WAY TO ACHIEVE YOUR ASPIRATIONS

Save your imagery from every enjoyable open water experience and use these memories in your triathlons. Recall them during race week and before the start.

MOTIVATIONAL THOUGHTS

Establish what motivates you and what scares you the most:

- What scares you most–racing against the clock, yourself or others?
- Do you like to be the hunted or lead from the front?

Once you know what type of athlete you are then you can unlock the key to a treasure trove full of personal records.

Most triathletes only have one strategy. They like to race against the clock and, if they are successful, they will beat their competitors, while others aim to be the best they can and improve on a previous performance. Most triathletes aim to compete against the rest of the field.

It is no good to be meticulous with your planning of every session, every route, specific race pace training, recovery pace for each workout, sticking within or below your heart rate zones for each training plan but then not think about how your mind will be acting.

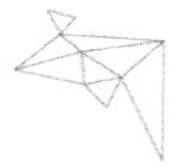

"All great achievements have one thing in common, people with a passion to succeed." Pat Cash

USING FEAR FOR PERFORMANCE

You need to be winning in the mind before you even consider competing in a triathlon. It's important to have a good clear mental vision with a strategy.

What are you driven by?

Do you like being hunted and being chased from behind, then use this fear to keep you going, make sure you stay in the moment and in control to keep an even pace, avoid going so hard that you have to slow down.

If you like chasing others make sure you pace yourself first in your mind, then during training and finally during your triathlon. Watch others ahead: if they're strong on the hills then ease up down the hills. Work out your game plan and when to attack and overtake them.

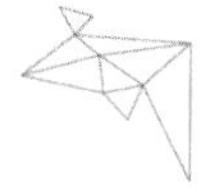

"I am prepared for the worse, but hope for the best."
Benjamin Disraeli

WINNERS AND RUNNERS-UP

WINNER OF THE MENTAL BATTLE

...is a person that achieves their goal. Their target time may actually be easy to achieve.

They may not be first overall to complete the triathlon or may not even win their age group or qualify for the world championships. They have effective coping strategies to achieve the best that they can.

RUNNER UP IN THE MENTAL BATTLE

A runner up is happy to concede first place and finish 2nd but this does not mean they are a loser. They are aware of their capabilities and will strive to improve and win in the future. They can also achieve greatness and have a long term objective.

USE THOUGHT PROCESSES IN EVERYDAY LIFE

We are a result of our values and what we believe. The mind dictates our thoughts and emotions.

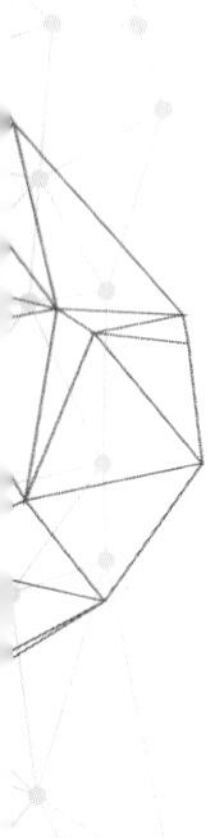

- Write down what you want to believe and this will help you believe.
- Read what you have written and this will reinforce your beliefs.
- Read out loud what you have written and you will hear what you believe.
- The more you think, see and hear, the greater your belief.
- When you believe, changes increase your positive self-belief.

Affirmations help us change:

1. Identify the negative thoughts and avoid negative self-talk.
2. Create affirmations to change negative thoughts.
3. Keep thinking more and more about these new positive affirmations.
4. Make sure you can believe these positive thoughts.
5. Be patient and enjoy the positive change that slowly occurs.

Examples include:

Instead of thinking:	Think:
'I cannot go fast in a triathlon.'	'I can go faster, it will just take time.'
'I cannot lose weight.'	'Lose a little bit each week and it all adds up.'
'Sports nutrition is so confusing.'	'If I practise I will soon find out what works best for me.'

MOTIVATION

Too much motivation can be detrimental

Delaying gratification is tough, but this will help during a competition when the urgency is to get to the finish line when the gun goes off! Do not compromise the long-term plan by starting too fast.

How to stay motivated—Keep mentally rehearsing previous great experiences or how proud were you when you overcame adversity.

HABITS

Negative Habits—How to change negative thoughts to positive

Put yourself in someone else's shoes, maybe someone who is older or slower or younger with less experience or physically challenged. Understand the importance of empathy.

You are always right if you learn from an experience and change your thoughts to improve next time.

Most people either do not like change or they find change stressful. Learn to embrace change for positive reasons.

Exercise will improve your feel good factor.

Take time out for yourself! Just for 10 minutes most days, do something that makes you feel good or happy.

Simple natural nutrition can change negative thoughts caused by simple sugars giving you highs and lows of blood sugar rushes. It will not only be a benefit to your health but your positive thoughts.

Catch up with friends and family, some studies have shown that a strong social network helps people live longer and healthier with a much more positive outlook on life.

All the above will help with a positive mind-set.

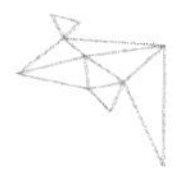

> **"I have not failed. I have just found 10,000 ways that won't work."**
> Thomas Alva Edison

Positive Habits–How to develop a 100% positive attitude

Remember: Doing triathlons is fun!

Believe in your ability!

The weather conditions (hot, cold, wind and rain) make the event a challenge for everyone.

Think positive thoughts!

Take responsibility for your own performance and let others be responsible for their result.

Be flexible with what can happen during a triathlon; then you will be in a much better position to cope with a performance.

Treat yourself as you would your best friend in the whole wide world.

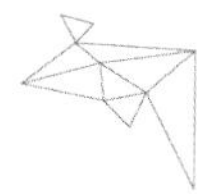

"It's kind of fun to do the impossible." Walt Disney

PRE-COMPETITION

In order to compete, it is important to be appropriately aroused and emotional. It will help if you know how to use these emotions, and if they are kept under control. Otherwise, they can prevent you from achieving your potential.

Positive emotions will make you more competitive.

Negative thoughts will cause you to think too much.

Lowering anxiety to the correct level will get you back on track mentally.

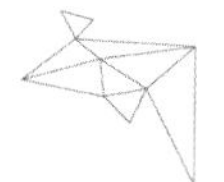

"There is nothing like first-hand evidence." Sherlock Holmes

What happens to the mind during a sporting event?

Every person has an opinion about everything, from a favorite color to the environment.

Athletes are no different when it comes to sport and what weather you prefer.

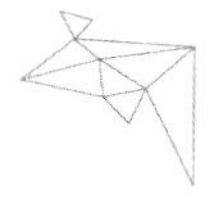

"Logic will get you from A to B. Imagination will take you everywhere." Albert Einstein

ANXIETY

Anxiety easily happens when the athlete does not have the capacity to deal with stress or that the stress is overwhelming. Anxiety causes fear, increases the heart and perspiration rates, and puts the mind in a stupor. This causes negative self-evaluations, expectations and thoughts of failure.

It is not all negative because anxiety is necessary for arousal.

Anxiety is made up of a mental (cognitive) component and a physiological (somatic) component. There is a direct link between them. Anxiety increases, performance increases and then it begins to decrease as anxiety continues to rise.

Emotions can either inhibit or inspire a great performance. Anxiety can increase and possibly overwhelm you. Instead of helping you, it can cause fear and mistakes to happen, creating even more anxiety. Without anxiety, you cannot stimulate your flight response, a necessary component of heightened athletic ability.

With anxiety, tension can occur. Manage this tension for a greater performance.

Recognize why and where you are tense.

Recognizing in advance when you are likely to become tense and mentally rephrasing will prevent tension from occurring by dealing with them before they become an issue.

When we imagine future feelings we find it impossible to ignore how we are feeling now. It is then impossible to think about our images of the future. Think about what makes you anxious head on and see it as one small negative compared to all your positive thoughts.

By repeatedly doing this, you will break the downward spiral of negativity.

By identifying your signature strengths, you reduce the amount of anxiety.

Most people have more imagined fears than actual fears. The best way to combat this is to think of a fear many times and make the outcome more and more favorable so it no longer makes you anxious. Otherwise, fears make us nervous, negatively affect decision making, and will change our behavior.

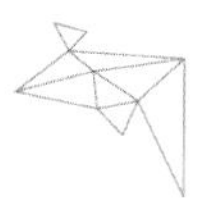

"Each success only buys an admission ticket to a more difficult problem." Henry Kissinger

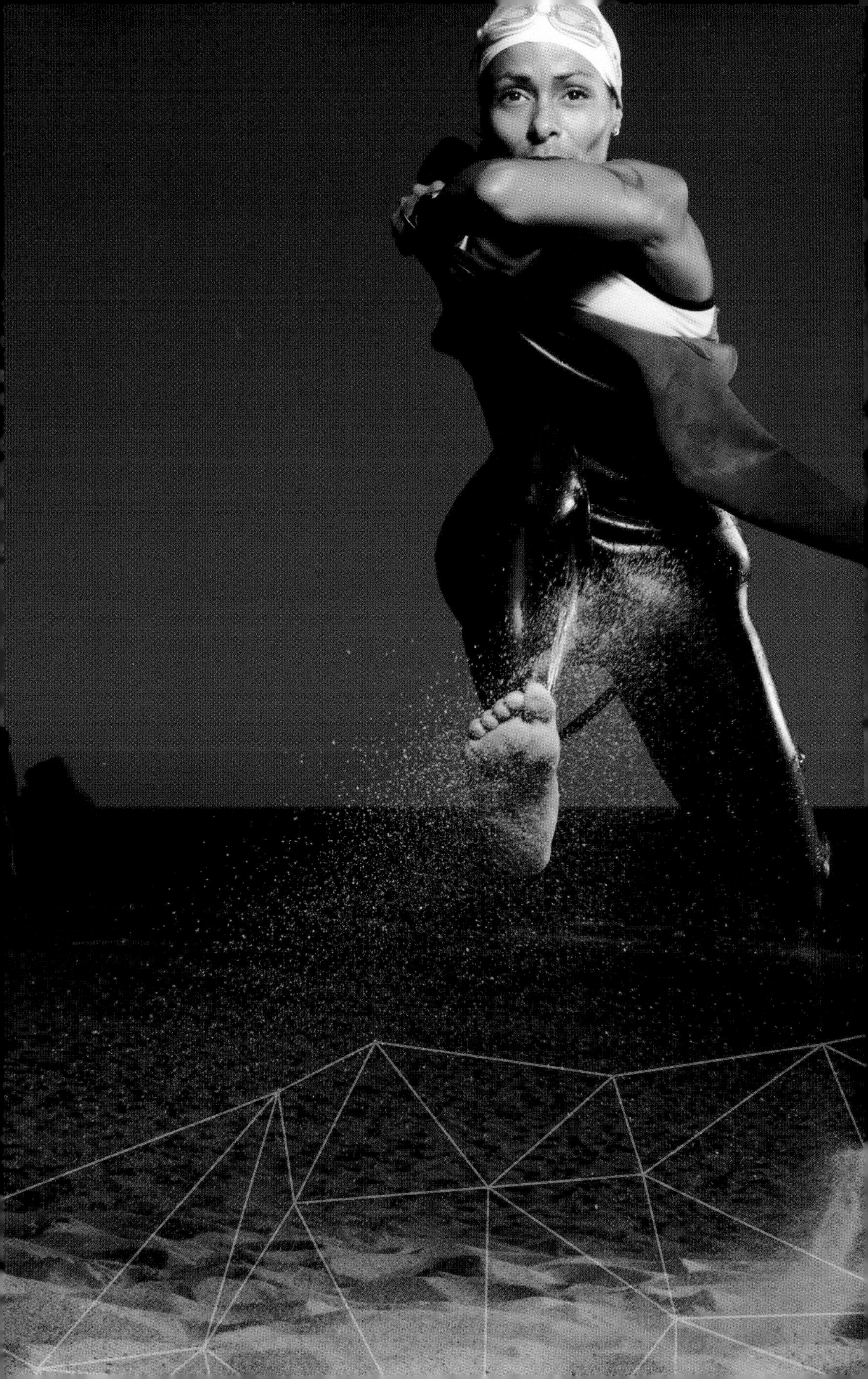

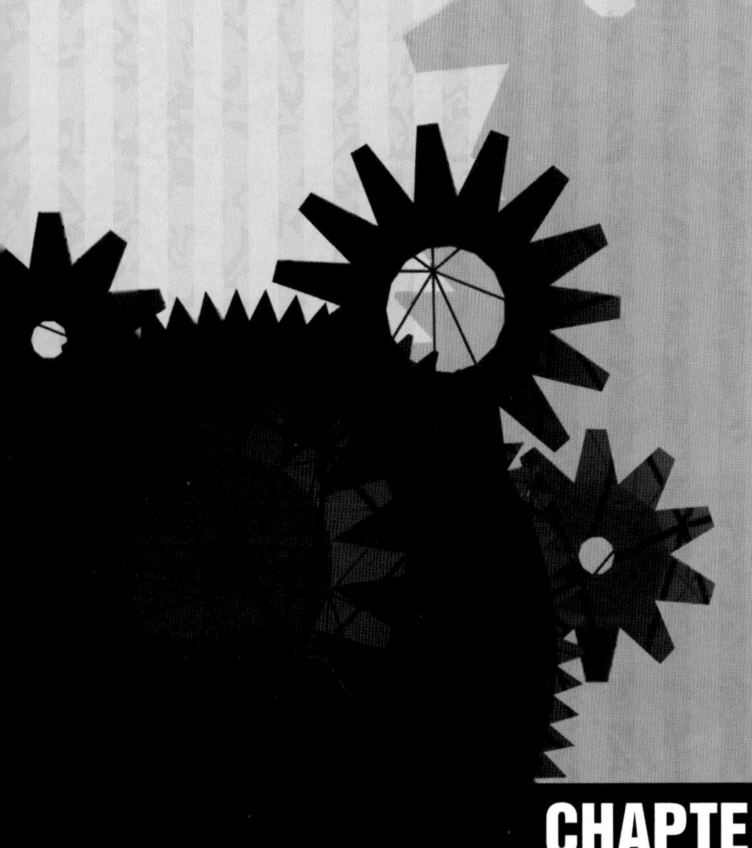

CHAPTER NINE.

TRIATHLETE'S MIND

TRIATHLETE'S MIND

Visualization on a regular basis (5 minutes each day) can really change you from lacking self-belief to becoming quietly confident. Creating a blueprint in your mind is like a street map of how to get from A to B.

Most people can put on a brave face and persona. Inner confidence can be achieved by almost everyone. The difference between the triathlete that fades at the end of a triathlon and the one that keeps going is all in the mind.

Lack of belief causes the following to happen:

- An inner feeling of not being fast or good enough.
- Extreme nerves before and at the start of your triathlon.
- You always have great training sessions but underperform during the triathlon.
- Ongoing negative thoughts that increase in frequency or severity the closer to your event.
- Always have problems sleeping the night before a competition.
- Forgetful race week.
- Forgetting to take items to the triathlon.
- Clumsy and making mistakes in transition—not laying out kit correctly, running in the wrong direction or not being able to find your bike.
- Being concerned with things that are unlikely to happen, like thinking you will forget to put on your helmet before running with your bike.
- Increasing dread of competing the closer you get to the triathlon.
- Repeating the same mistakes at every triathlon.

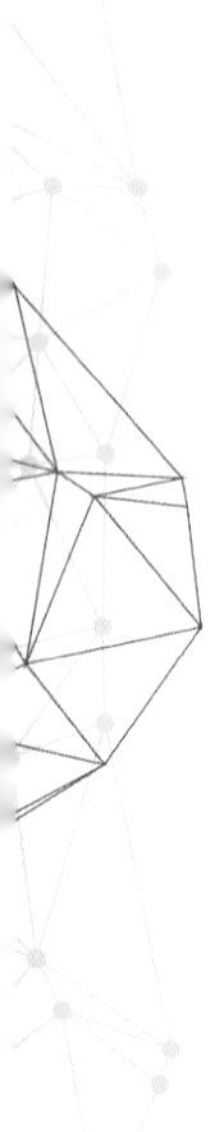

Believing is achieving–the more confident you become the more you reduce anxiety and all its symptoms.

Having some fear and trepidation is perfectly normal so do not get nervous if you feel nervous.

Visualized daily will instills belief and greater control on triathlon day.

DAILY VISUALIZATION

Every day for just 5 minutes all you have to do is imagine the perfect triathlon in your mind. Think about the course, the air temperature, the noise, and seeing other competitors as though you are actually competing. Now you have the best race you want to happen, and can feel the elation and amazing experience. Repeat this daily and it will be ingrained into your subconscious mind.

Now it is time to think about little unlikely issues that may occur. You get a flat tire 2 miles from the finish of your triathlon. Remaining positive in your mind will help you stay relaxed so you can think in a calm way about what you would do–either slow down and carry on or change it. Not finishing is not an option, so get back into the feel-good visualization of the perfect race you have been repeating and finish strongly.

The more of these little scenarios you consider the more you will feel confident with your ability. Your confidence levels will gradually improve, and you will sleep much better the night before your triathlon.

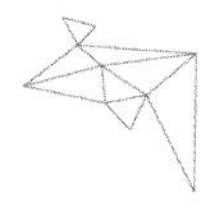

"The brave man is not he who does not feel afraid, but he who conquers that fear." Nelson Mandela

Benefits of daily triathlon visualization include:

- These daily thoughts will keep you motivated
- Learn to deal with anxiety during race week and on triathlon day
- Improve technical aspects of swimming, cycling and running

- Learn new skills, like removing wet suit quicker
- Going into autopilot, moving smoothly and relaxed through transition
- Remind yourself to be relaxed during a triathlon
- Overcome fear and nerves
- Quickly overcome any negativity during training and racing
- Remain more positive about the triathlon each day
- Increase your daily enthusiasm to train
- Allow yourself to go into autopilot with nutrition and hydration
- Learn to embrace the triathlon
- Become less intimidated by other competitors
- Allow yourself to not worry about others and their criticism
- Ignore others who cheat by drafting
- Self-belief will increase considerably
- Dramatically improve your confidence the closer you get to race day
- Relax much easier and quicker once you start competing
- Banish negativity and maintain a positive attitude
- Reduce the uncertainty of the uncontrollable
- Less stress can speed up recovery from training
- Speed up recovering from illness and sickness
- You are more likely to be proactive at dealing with injuries rather than doing nothing
- Sort out issues much easier if they occur during the triathlon
- Sleep much better and wake up feeling like you have solved a problem and there is nothing to worry about
- More likely to find creative ways to train when life gets in the way
- Being more patient in everyday life and persistent with your training

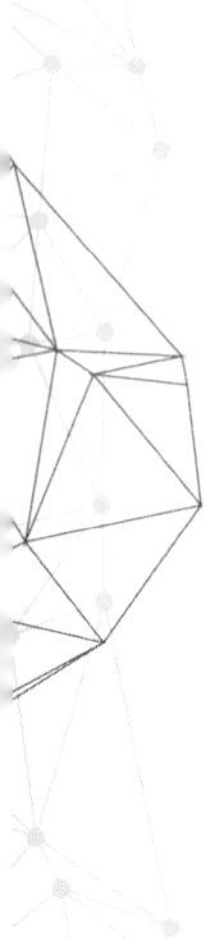

- Greatly improve your chances of success even during adversity
- Learn to make contact with the sleeping giant inside you—your subconscious
- Squash your fears and concerns on a daily basis

PRE-TRIATHLON THOUGHTS

Think about your thoughts and feelings in the final days before a triathlon.

What goes through your mind the day before your triathlon or waking up race morning? How do your emotions change 10 minutes before the start? Self-talk will make you far more optimistic of a favorable outcome. Tell yourself enough times and you will believe it!

Thoughts and words we think or say affect our emotions, especially in the 5-10 minutes before your triathlon.

What separates two people in a triathlon by a small margin is all in the mind.

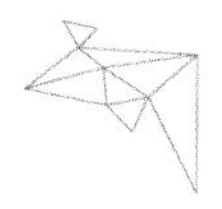

> **"In any situation, the best thing you can do is the right thing; the next best thing you can do is the wrong thing; the worst thing you can do is nothing."** Theodore Roosevelt

If you doubt the strength of the mind then consider the more relaxed you are or the more experience you have, the better your performance. Experience can be recovered from the library of memories stored away in your subconscious mind.

Every swimming, cycling, running or triathlon session is stored, ready to be used when you need it.

It is very common for triathletes to finish a race in their predicted time no matter what happened on race day. They trained the body and mind to get to the finish line as planned.

The triathlete that made the least mistakes is often the winner; they had mentally rehearsed the triathlon and had fewer doubts. If you think you are going to make a mistake, you are telling your body to make the mistake. It is like whispering to yourself. A positive thought is likely to give a favorable outcome and a negative thought is likely to end in a negative result.

Positive people are not luckier; they just have positive thoughts. If you have negativity then you need to clear your mind and focus again.

Repeating a few positive words or statements many times each day and in the 10 minutes before the start will reprogram positive thoughts and push away negative thoughts.

An affirmation or mantra is a technique that has been used by sportsmen and women all around the world. An example of an affirmation could be "smooth and strong" or "be efficient and save energy."

You can use the same words for swim, bike, run or have different ones, for example for swim you could use "long and powerful," for the bike "spin smoothly" and the run section of the triathlon "fast leg turnover." Some triathletes even have different sayings for different distances.

Try to avoid words that can cause anxiety like "fast and furious" unless of course that works for you. One triathlete I knew who raced sprint triathlons changed her mantra and this reduced her over-striding, which resulted in her running much faster.

Some mantras are private and others are known to the world. Muhammad Ali's famous saying was "I am the greatest." Not only did this make him know he was the greatest but it also told every other boxer in the world he was.

Your own mantra must give you confidence.

Rather than saying, "Come on, you will do it," try "Come on, you can do it."

Make sure it gives a lift and picks you up mentally.

I find that an affirmation that is in tune with your movements can get you to keep exact timing. Triathletes that train to music should consider humming a tune because most triathlons do not allow you to listen to music while competing. First start humming while listening to music, and then hum without the music.

Using music for your optimum swim stroke cycle, cadence and strides per minute means you should have 3 tunes in your head or mantras—one for swim, bike and run.

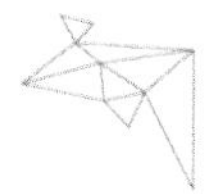

"**Great minds think alike, they first have a thought then carry out a calculated action.**" Mark Kleanthous

POST-TRIATHLON BLUES

POST MIND BLUES

You need to rest to allow your body to recover and also to allow you to clear your mind.

Mild depression can be a sign that you need to recharge the mind from competition and information over load. Nutrition can also cause the same symptoms or exacerbate the problem if you have had a low sugar diet (cakes, white sugar on cereals, tea, coffee, jams, marmalades and honey on bread). If, after a competition, you have sugar, your body may react because it is now super sensitive. This ultimately affects your mood swings.

Recovery is when the body can super compensate and the mind can learn from your recent past sporting experience.

Signs of triathlon blues:

- You are missing the challenge of training for a triathlon.
- You have a feeling of something missing in life.
- Everything seems an effort.
- You may experience sadness.
- You have more time now due to not training every spare moment.
- Mood swings as a result of procrastination after thinking of your triathlon.
- Bored—plenty of time on your hands.

- Total loss of direction and a feeling of despondency.
- No direction or real purpose.
- Mood like depression is a sign you have not fully overcome how you could have improved your performance in training or during the triathlon.

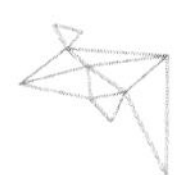

"The only way to prove that you're good at sport is to lose."
Ernie Banks

THINGS TO CONSIDER AFTER YOUR TRIATHLON

You must take time off from thinking about your triathlon, otherwise you will delay your enthusiasm for returning.

Expect to have "flashbacks" or "what if" questions whizzing inside your head.

"I wish I had kept to my nutrition plan then I would not have had to walk."

"I should have paced myself better." "Why did I borrow a pair of new wheels that did not work on race day?" "I should have used a special needs bag."

Avoid thinking of the past and instead learn from your experience and use this in the future.

Your body needs a break and so does your mind.

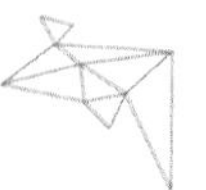

"Adversity causes some men to break, others to break records."
William Arthur Ward

A cloudy mind can be a sign that you have post-race bleakness, which can involve the following symptoms:

- Short-term memory loss.
- Using the wrong words or names or getting them mixed up. For example, you might say "bridge under water" instead of saying "bridge over water."

- Inability to organize your thoughts.
- Poor concentration.
- Disturbed sleep from a restless body. You are not tired from exercise but your mind is very active.

There is no set pattern but expect the phase to happen like this.

YOUR MIND AFTER YOUR TRIATHLON

First stage—post-race 0-14 days—Euphoria and lots of positive thoughts.

Second stage—post-race 3-21 days—Sense of achievement mixed up with flashbacks of what could you have done better. Positive and negative thoughts all mixed up.

Third stage—14 days-2 years—Mostly lows with a few highs in emotion. Very few middle-range emotions.

WHAT YOU CAN DO

Think about the positives not the negatives. You are now part of a very elite group of people who have competed in a triathlon. You cannot change the race result, but provided you have learned something, you can move on.

The absence of anticipation and excitement has now gone and you are back at work. Find a new enjoyable thing to do.

Without adequate switch-off time, you will fail to let the mind recover.

Below are some symptoms you may experience post-race during the next 2 years:

- Grumpiness—more than usual.
- Sadness—like you have lost a best friend.
- Boredom—plenty of time on your hands or you are simply wasting time.
- Restlessness—you are still not ready to resume training.
- Sudden mood swings—often as a result of earlier procrastination.

- Not motivated—even to do things you would normally enjoy.
- The loss of any direction will result in feelings of aimlessness and despondency.
- You feel you are missing something to train for.
- Gloominess is a sign that you are missing training.
- Skin problems (the largest organ in the body) are a mirror image of our insides.
- Despondency—everything is an effort, but you should not be tired.
- Melancholy—little things that do not normally bother you now annoy you.
- Clumsiness—a sign you are still thinking about the triathlon.

Don't ignore feelings but listen to your mind and think about what you have achieved rather than what you wanted to achieve.

Exercise can help with mood swings so think of trying a new sport.

HOW TO BEAT THE POST-RACE BLUES

You have devoted a lot of time and effort to fit in training, but now you do not need to.

You should expect to feel lost and empty for up to 24 months after giving up triathlons.

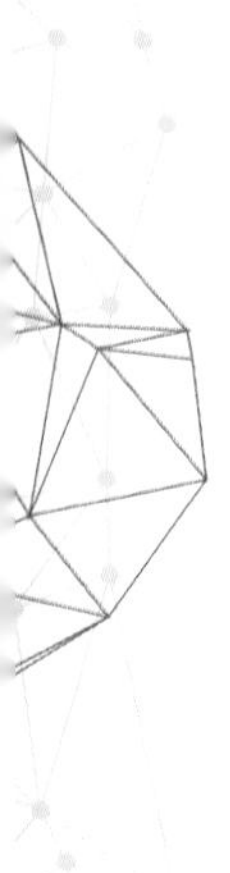

YOU

- "You" have the same dedication but now have no target.
- "You" have determination but no triathlon-produced endorphins.
- "You" still have drive but no huge purpose.
- "You" have more free time than before but no short-term goal.

What you do next is important in order to beat the post-triathlon blues.

Avoid thinking about what might have been. Write down the whole race and what you learned. How good was your pace, nutrition and non-competitive mind?

Add to the list as you recall the triathlon in your mind.

Making notes will stop your mind from questioning yourself.

Many triathletes appear to suffer after their major triathlon or when they retire from sports.

It has been said that sportsmen die twice—the first time is after they retire.

Dedicating your life to preparing and then competing causes a huge gap in your life after a triathlon.

Making personal sacrifices to achieve the best you can during a competition can be hard to cope with if you are not pleased with the outcome.

Two triathletes sprint to the finish line; the first across the post may be disappointed because the triathlon did not go according to plan.

The second in the sprint finish may be pleased with a particular finishing time. It could be a lifetime best and they exceeded their expectations.

Without the routine of training and no adrenaline being released due to not training and competing, your body feels that there is something missing.

Now the mind is no longer being kept busy; it has time to ponder on wishing you had achieved greater things.

Many athletes can deal with the day-to-day training stress and then race day pressure, but now they miss this part of the preparing and competing in a triathlon.

Some athletes are pleased to stop due to the intense pressure they put on themselves, and some even consider that it had been a burden to train and that they are now relieved to have stopped training for a triathlon.

What most triathletes have in common when they give up sport or get to the end of the season is a feeling of emptiness.

A de-training of the body and mind should happen after a major triathlon rather than stopping completely.

Severe depression occurs in some age groups and professional athletes in all sports, including athletics, boxing, cricket, football and swimming. There are a lot of famous people who have publicly discussed their depression after quitting sport. In many instances, they have attempted suicide and some have resulted in death.

It is likely that due to the Internet, including Twitter and Facebook, more athletes have become more famous than ever before, so when they retire the loss can be greater.

This has filtered down to some age group triathletes who are Internet heroes and have to broadcast their every physical movement all over social media.

Recently, I read on twitter:

"What a waste of time. I went to the gym earlier and forgot to tweet it."

It is perfectly natural to have a profound sense of loss when you do not have a focus for training.

Stages of depression and thinking of making a comeback are common for every person in every sport, especially in triathlon where it attracts highly motivated single-minded individuals.

You experience a loss of identity once you are no longer training for triathlons.

To be successful in sport, a sort of tunnel vision is required. Once you take that away, there is nothing left to focus on.

Exercise causes serotonin to be released, so stopping training will reduce this level, which can then cause depression. More studies need to be carried out to compare levels of competitive and retired triathletes.

WHAT CAN A PROFESSIONAL OR AGE GROUP TRIATHLETE DO TO OVERCOME POST-RACE BLUES?

When you prepared for the triathlon it is likely that you were fitter, not necessarily healthier, but happy.

Find things to make you laugh and smile. Spend that mental energy in other interests or new hobbies. Learn how to cope with stress now that you are not exercising. Do things you never had time to do during your training, such as home improvements and getting in touch with friends.

Post-race depression is not often seen even by close loved ones and is even harder for the triathlete to identify.

There is also a darker side after sport. Most triathletes appear to be happier with their lives when they were non-stop at 100%, living and training for a triathlon than now when they are at only 85% and have nothing to train for.

Triathletes revel in the frenetic 24/7 hugely ambitious lifestyle of training, working, eating and sleeping. When this all stops they appear not to be as satisfied with their lives.

More research needs to be carried out if effective coping strategies during sport can help prevent or reduce post-competition depression. There does not appear to be a direct correlation between the length of post-competition blues, or the severity of withdrawal symptoms and the length of time someone has been involved in the sport.

Too many factors, like an injury, can cut a sporting career short. Also was there already a long-term plan for not competing after the triathlon, and whether the triathlon achieved your aims and ambitions?

Finding something else to fill the gap left by a triathlon will be a start to overcoming life's problems until next time.

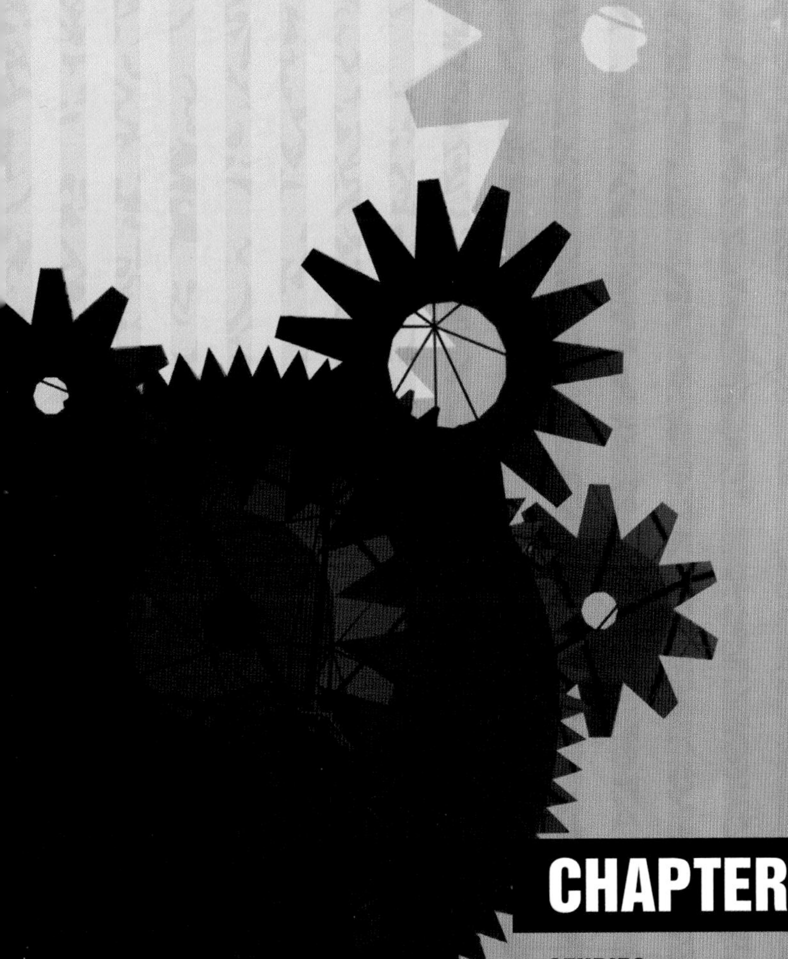

CHAPTER TEN.

STUDIES

TEN.

STUDIES

This chapter looks at research that explains how the mind helps you win or lose, give in or finish.

To compete in a triathlon, you have to overcome physical and psychological issues, so you need effective coping strategies. This will make it both enjoyable and will considerably increase your chances of success. For many triathletes, the biggest challenge is not the distance or the pace; it's what goes on inside a 6-inch space within your own head.

External environmental factors are referred to as "stressors" and reactions to external stressors are referred to as "stress."

Stressors can cause anxiety stress, which will be debilitating to sporting performance. Below are some useful real-life scenarios to help you in the future.

The skill is in appraising a situation as stressful without it causing you stress. The same stressor will be either perceived as a nuisance or challenging, depending on if you have considered the situation already in your mind or have experienced it in the past. New issues never considered before are likely to be classified as stressors if you feel they are out of your control, but mental rehearsal imagery can switch this problem to being challenging instead.

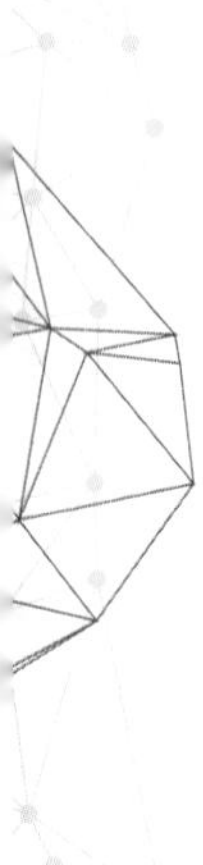

If the triathlete interprets a situation as not stressful or of slight concern, then a coping strategy may not be required.

There has been minimal research into race stressors on triathletes and how to overcome problems with effective coping strategies. One study by Buman, et al., 2008, explored how to implement effective strategies to overcome adversity among active non-elite endurance triathletes. This was done with detailed interviews before and as soon as possible after their triathlon.

The findings revealed the most frequently anticipated race stressors listed here in no particular order.

They were mechanical and equipment failure, injury, environmental factors, the initial leg of the triathlon, the swim start, and nutrition and hydration. Yet the most saliently reported acute stressors were injury, environmental factors, the racecourse itself, the behavior of other athletes, and exhaustion.

The triathletes in the study had no strategy or a wide range of coping strategies before or during the triathlon.

The most successful triathletes have a multi-pronged vision of getting to the finish line. They have already worked out in their minds what may go wrong from past sporting experiences or learning from others. In their minds they have many race day scenarios and "what-ifs" for emergency action procedures.

At the end of this chapter you will find an interesting study carried out and completed in 2013 by multiple Ironman® finisher, Peter Hayward, titled Coping Strategies: Selection and Effectiveness in Relation to Anticipated and Acute Race Stressors Encountered by Non-Elite Long-Distance Male Triathletes.

This study will help you have a better understanding of why mental rehearsal is not just something else to do but a necessary requirement for sporting excellence.

Multi-dimensional coping strategy is a mental and physical struggle, and you should have an action plan worked out in your mind. It needs to be self-regulatory and flexible to alter your thinking behavior, which will need to change with the environment.

For example, if during a triathlon it has been unexpectedly hot and as a result you have not been hydrating enough, you will now experience thirst sensations and your emergency action plan needs to get into action as soon as possible.

First, you need to slow down to be able to absorb your fluid, and you need to know how much to drink. But understand that if you ignore the early warning signs of not drinking enough, you could experience cramps or become so dehydrated that you do not finish. Failure to hydrate will result in a physiological slow down and psychological turmoil thus increasing negative thoughts. This will then result in not being able to keep up at the current pace.

Mood swings can happen from becoming low on energy and even small drops in hydration levels, so make decisions on the information available and try to avoid worrying about things that are not in your control.

Many different things can happen during your build-up and during the triathlon to limit your racing performance. Being flexible and adapting to the circumstances in a positive and constructive way will help you have the best race possible. Occasionally experience partial dehydration in training so you can act upon the warning signs. Some triathletes experience dehydration for the first time in a triathlon and either ignore the symptoms or do not recognize what is happening until it is too late because they did not associate the signs with the need to drink more.

IT'S THE THOUGHT THAT COUNTS

You have the chance to be awesome by taking control of your thoughts.

Having effective coping strategies in your armory will also improve confidence. You can make matters worse by thinking about a problem and not finding a solution, so it becomes an issue in your mind.

Different coping strategies can be used by different individuals with the same success rate.

You should have an effective coping strategy for every possible scenario, anything that is ominous or is likely to avoid you achieving your desires.

Anticipated coping strategies (before triathlon day) are ones you have personally experienced, thought about, or learned from other triathletes, books, or the Internet. This could be your goggles leak. You have already tried this in training, making them stop leaking in the pool, clearing and replacing them back on your face, then try this skill in open water. If and when this happens in a triathlon, you will instantly remove the goggles, replace them and carry on without a care in the world. Anything that can be practiced physically as well as mentally should be done to reinforce your library of mental imagery.

Actual coping strategies (during triathlon day) include dealing with a situation using a combination of mental rehearsal techniques, including thinking clearly under a stressful situation. You are struggling to remove your cycle helmet after dismounting and racking your bike. You simply hold your breath, close your mouth, unclip the buckle, remove the helmet, put on your shoes and run to the exit.

A coping strategy is making a conscious effort to alleviate the stress associated with it and overcoming the distraction. This could be physical or mental or a combination, and can go head-to-head with an emotion or seeking a distraction thought to tag it to.

An effective coping strategy of the mind can be your biggest asset or your worst enemy.

First you have to appraise the situation, then deal with either a coping strategy, a problem-focused action plan, or a combination of both.

A coping strategy addresses the situation with a reaction, while an effective action plan deals completely with the problem to allow for the desired outcome.

EXAMPLE—EMOTION COPING TRIATHLON STRATEGY

In this scenario, you have to manage your emotional response to stress by being optimistic, smiling, and thinking positively of reaching the finishing line. Another alternative is the denial of the situation and thinking of something else you would enjoy doing.

Your mood has changed from aiming for a fast time to just finishing. Assessing that you have been falling behind with your calorie intake has led to a dip in your performance and a fall in your blood sugar level, resulting in a downward mood swing. By concentrating on having enough calories, but not too many, you will soon recover and get back to your desired pace and feel a lot more positive.

EXAMPLE—PROBLEM-SOLVING STRATEGY

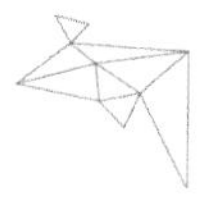

„An inconvenience is only an adventure wrongly considered; an adventure is an inconvenience rightly considered.“
Gilbert Keith Chesterton

In this scenario, you have to alter your actions to help you achieve your potential. Below are two examples:

Example 1—You are about 35 minutes from the finish line of your triathlon, and your concern is getting the stitch if you eat or drink something, then pushing hard to the finishing line.

You need to recall how many calories you have had and listen to your body for any signs of fatigue. Then, and only then, decide if you need calories for energy from a gel or just electrolytes to prevent cramps, or just water or nothing, and then push to the finish line.

Example 2—It is really hot so instead of taking the shortest legal route, you choose to run on the course in the shade until you cool down.

It is important to do a regular checkup from head to toe for any signs of tightness, areas that are rubbing, if you are feeling cold or running low on energy levels, and how you have been recently performing with the competition to make effective coping strategies work. Just because you are maintaining your position with others, you still may be slowing. Get back on track with nutrition and watch yourself start passing others.

Avoid ignoring a small problem that could get considerably worse.

For example, your skin is starting to burn before you complete the bike segment, so you quickly rub on sunblock before the run, allowing yourself to cool down in the marquee before tackling the run. Do not ignore your instincts to save a few seconds in transition. You may regret it, and it will distract you later during the run.

You can turn a major stressor into a minor concern by dealing with it quickly.

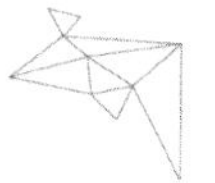

"Our greatest weakness lies in giving up. The most certain way to succeed is always to try just one more time." Thomas A Edison.

FEED STATION STRESSOR

Example—you drop a drink bottle at a feed station and decide to continue. You assessed the situation and realize you still have enough fluid until the next feed station or the end of the bike run. Make your decision and stick by it until you cross the finish line, then consider whether it a good idea or not. I have observed this happening to others and because they were focusing on regretting their mistake instead of hydrating, they ended up getting to the next feed station with some fluid in their bottle that they should really have drank.

BIKE STRESSOR

Having a well-rehearsed plan in your head of how to fix a puncture while relaxed is no good in the following situations:

1—If you only mentally rehearse changing a flat tire and you never physically change a tire, or never change it under pressure. Once competent at changing a tire, time yourself changing it in the quickest time possible. Consider a head-to-head session changing a tire with a friend for fun, which will cause a little fun pressure.

2—You experience three punctures and you only have two spare inner tubes.

The effectiveness of a coping strategy is reducing negativity or overcoming a problem that allows the triathlete to continue and complete the triathlon in the best possible time.

The relationship between stress and a coping strategy is that it has been tried and tested hundreds of times in your mind. In many situations, mental practice can keep you from freezing with fear.

Men and women both have strategies to overcome possible problems. Women tend to use emotion-focused techniques more than men, who use problem-focused strategies.

TRIATHLON STRESSORS INCLUDE:

- Injury
- Mental errors
- Physical errors
- Psychological demands
- Competitive worries
- Anxiety
- Self-doubt

ENVIRONMENTAL STRESSORS INCLUDE:

- Heat
- Cold
- Wind
- Terrain
- Altitude
- Hydration
- Distance
- Sleep problems
- Rain
- Equipment failure

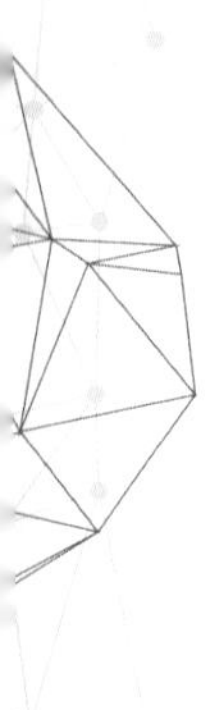

Triathlon-specific stressors can be anticipated based on the experience of the athlete.

Expect the unexpected. Mild stressors or disastrous situations might happen, so be prepared to expect the unexpected and you will be able to deal with them. It's a natural response to deal with anything unexpected as being more of a threat.

Once you are comfortable with each individual mental image, combine two together, like sweat (salt) in your eye and a blister developing. Pouring water on your face may alleviate the eye but the discomfort from the blister may get worse. Spending just 5-10 seconds on mental imagery about coping with a blister is unlikely to be sufficient to have effective coping strategies. You can think about walking to tend to your eye and this may temporarily alleviate the blister. The longer the event the more you may endure a problem, but the more time that you can take control of the situation the better the outcome will be.

If you have mentally rehearsed on a regular basis, then the greater the success that effective coping strategy will have on the performance. Having competed in 36 Ironman®, double Ironman® and triple Ironman® events, I have gone into autopilot when an issue has arisen and dealt with it like a robot without emotion. This is also efficient from an energy point of view.

An adult human brain requires about 12 watts or 20% of the power of a standard 60-watt light bulb. The brain weighs about 1.4 kg or about 2% of total body weight, but requires 20% of our resting metabolic rate (RMR). Neurons within the brain communicate with each other, even during sleep, to repair and rebuild themselves. It is likely that using mental imagery, rather than having to think, will require less energy for thinking and therefore you will have more time for moving forward.

The details below are based on real-life experiences backed up by effective coping strategies.

10.1 STRATEGIES

MENTAL IMAGERY, IF DONE ENOUGH TIMES, CAN END UP FEELING REALISTIC.

MECHANICAL / EQUIPMENT FAILURE

Mechanical–Swimming goggles steaming up, gears not working on your bike.

Equipment failure–Swimming goggles strap snapping just before the start, chain or handlebar breaking, bike computer not working or heart rate monitor not receiving heart rate data, bike cables not working, rear mechanism derailleur and gears not working, punctures and not being able to fix them.

Your bike may have been damaged while travelling to the triathlon. Arriving with adequate time for an overseas triathlon or knowing if the organizations have a bike mechanic onsite is worth knowing beforehand.

I have known many competitors who have travelled by air to a triathlon and their bike has been delayed, and it was touch and go if the bike would arrive in time for the triathlon. There is only so much you can do to get your bike in time. Knowing your bike measurements and carrying your race kit on board to limit the problems associated with using different clothing, bike and run shoes will reduce the risk if you have to borrow a bike for the triathlon.

PHYSICAL EFFECTIVE COPING STRATEGY TO REDUCE ANXIETY

Have a strategy to help reduce pre-race and race-day anxiety.

Do a bike service four weeks before the triathlon and replace gear and brake cables along with checking and tightening bolts. Ask the mechanic to check if anything needs attention. Don't leave it until race week as they may be too busy to check your bike, and if they do find something that needs replacing, the part may not arrive in time, which will cause anxiety before and during your triathlon. There are only two things worse than training with a bike that may not be 100% reliable, and that is competing in a triathlon and wishing you had taken the bike to a specialist sooner to get it fixed. The worst scenario is the bike is unreliable and does not allow you to complete your triathlon.

Get new tires fitted three weeks before race day to make sure there is no problem with the tires or inner tubes.

Six to two weeks before your triathlon do a final race route check. If possible, first drive the cycle route then cycle it. Depending on the run route, you can run or cycle (road or MTB) the run course.

The more familiar you are with the course the better; don't fret if they change the course at the last minute as everyone will be in the same position.

When checking out the bike route, look for potholes (they can cause flat tires or force bottles to be lost), ride the toughest hills and look for any sudden surprises like drain covers or poor road surfaces as you go around corners.

If you can cycle up a hill in training, it will give you a lot of confidence during the final preparation phase, and give you plenty of time to think during your taper. You will have a positive mindset of your ability on the course on race day. Cycling up a hill in practice will teach you how to pace yourself up a hill thus saving energy for the run.

For a technical event, get a friend to take you to the top of a hill and practice descending or practice a particular section that you are concerned with.

During the triathlon run reconnaissance, establish what type of shoes you need. If the conditions change due to heavy rain, will you need off-road shoes? Look for potholes, where to conserve energy before a hill, and be observant for tree roots and holes that could cause an injury during the run.

MUSCULAR PROBLEMS LIKE CRAMPS, HAMSTRINGS, SPASMS, OR CALF TIGHTNESS

Learn how much you can push yourself in training and when to back off a little. Then push yourself again so you can dial in just the right amount of effort on triathlon day.

MENTAL COPING STRATEGY TO REDUCE ANXIETY

During a triathlon, you need to have technical, tactical and behavioral skills to improve performance and success.

Every time you improve these skills, save the memory with a smile.

Confronting problems by thinking directly about the problem or dissociation can be equally as successful.

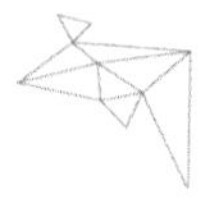

" **Optimism is the faith that leads to achievement. Nothing can be done without hope and confidence.**" Helen Keller

KNOW THE TRIATHLON COURSE

If you have driven or ridden the course, you can then mentally rehearse the event in your mind. If you have cycled the bike route, try and visualize the wind on your face, when you have a tailwind, and when you have a headwind to push you along fast.

Having a mental rehearsal of the route, knowing when to eat and drink and what gears to use for each part of the course makes the unknown known, resulting in improved mental fortitude.

Environmental Factors

Train in all weather conditions—hot, cold, dry, humid, calm, rain, fast days and windy days—so that whatever triathlon day throws your way you have experienced it many times before.

For example, cold morning swims, a hot midday sun beating down during a bike ride, mid-afternoon humid running and cool evenings. Judge your pace, alter your hydration and nutrition strategy, wear appropriate clothing based on the conditions, and be flexible with changing weather conditions.

THE SWIM'S MOST COMMON ANXIETIES EXPERIENCED

Mass start swimming, getting bumped in the triathlon swim, goggles being knocked off, or your wetsuit coming undone.

Swimming in cold water, overheating, not being able to see ahead due to the mist, blinded by the rising sun, being kicked at the turn buoys, swimming against a current and in a straight line in waves.

All can be overcome by practice, practice, practice in many different situations, including open water swim competitions or replicated with friends swimming in close proximity.

Give a friend a slight lead in an open water swim, practice working out and try to follow them. Make them zigzag so you have to keep looking up to practice your sighting skills.

Practice fast swimming around a buoy or swim around a friend who is treading water, then take turns and get constructive feedback on how you can improve.

COLD WATER STRATEGY

Coping with cold water. During the swim, wear a latex, then a neoprene, then a race swim cap to reduce heat loss. Take frequent cold showers and baths and remember these experiences during these cold practice sessions so you will be better prepared on race morning. Wash your face with cold water rather than warm water every day and remind yourself why you are doing it.

A warm breakfast like oatmeal plus a warm drink like coffee will warm you up inside and will help before a cold triathlon swim. Keep warm by wearing a warm hat on top of your swim cap so you don't get cold before the swim start, and don't forget to remove the hat before getting into the water. Dry yourself after a swim. Yes, I know it is a triathlon and you will lose 5 seconds with a quick rub of the towel, but it could save 200 calories by not using body heat to keep you warm.

Wear clothing that is quick drying without causing you to sweat because this will keep you warm. Even consider using socks and overshoes, etc.

OVERHEATING IN THE TRIATHLON SWIM

Overheating in the swim can be prevented by a method known as gulping in water by pulling the wetsuit away from your neck. Avoid undoing the wetsuit neck, but allow water to get inside your wetsuit while swimming. I have done this drafting behind another swimmer and only lost a small distance, and within 2 strokes was back drafting.

BEING ABLE TO SEE WHERE YOU ARE GOING WHILE SWIMMING

Try to have 2 pairs of swimming goggles (clear and tinted) and decide which pair to use on race morning. Both are likely to be a compromise–the clear pair are great when you start because as the sun comes up you may become blinded by its rays or the glare from the water's surface. A tinted pair may be too dark when you start but then ideal when the sun's glare becomes stronger. Few triathlon swims are point-to-point so you are likely to swim into the sun's glare during your triathlon.

COPING STRATEGY FOR FEAR OF THE DARK DEPTHS BELOW

Use a pair of tinted goggles in the swimming pool to experience what it is like not being able to see the bottom in open water.

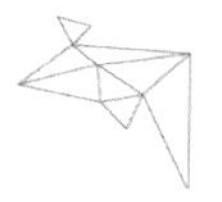

"You drown not by falling into the river, but by staying submerged in it." Paulo Coelho

STRAIGHT LINE SWIMMING STRATEGY

If your swimming pool has lanes for swimming alongside a fun session, get used to swimming in wavy water inside before venturing out into open water to swim in waves.

Practice sighting to help you swim in a straight line while swimming in smooth, flat water, then progress to swimming in rough water so it becomes second nature on triathlon day.

OVERCOME ANXIETY LOSING SWIM GOGGLES

Place your swim goggle strap under your swim cap so if they get knocked off, you are unlikely to lose them completely because they will still be attached to your head. I have competed in more than 460 triathlons and have never lost a pair of goggles yet using this strategy.

APPREHENSIVE ABOUT YOUR ABILITY COMPARED TO OTHERS AROUND YOU

Swim start–Make friends with those next to you, wish them good luck, then tell them what your projected swim time will be. Ask them so you can make a decision during the swim to draft, take it in turns, let them go or overtake and push harder. If you're faster, most times they will let you get in front of them before the start.

CONCERNED ABOUT RACE DAY MELTDOWN

I have spoken to hundreds of triathletes after their disappointing races and the majority blamed slowing down, walking or not finishing due to lack of time to train. What was obvious to me was their poor performances were mostly due to not having the correct number of calories and not having a timeline nutrition plan. Not one person who has taken my advice has been disappointed in future competitions. Finally, by having a meticulous tried and tested nutrition plan, you can avoid this disappointment.

HYDRATION TRIED AND TESTED STRATEGY

Having the correct amount of hydration and nutrition to avoid gastrointestinal or stomach problems or slowing down from not enough calories is not an art, it's all about adjusting to what works for you in different conditions.

Train at race pace and ingest the planned calories to establish exactly what you can handle and how it helps you. Just like an actor or actress, you must have rehearsed a tried and tested strategy months before so you can fine tune it and know exactly what you are doing at least 6 weeks before your triathlon.

Remember to try nothing new on race day. Don't grasp at straws. You are simply taking a chance by grabbing onto something that is likely to be worthless. Stick to what you know. Race day is not the time to try something new—never ever experiment during your triathlon unless it is the last resort.

Avoid the common mistake of thinking twice as much food will be rocket fuel as too many calories can be worse than not enough and will lead to a digestive disaster.

SLOWING DOWN AND NEGATIVE THOUGHTS

An effective coping strategy to combat fatigue is to slow down. Yes, I know this is not what you want to read. Don't delay but snack little and often, let your body absorb the calories and soon you will be flying again and naturally speeding up. Positive self-talk will help reduce negative thoughts and allow you to concentrate on the here and now. Firstly, accept the situation then focus on what you need to do now.

Swim techniques—If your arms are fatigued during the swim, take slightly shorter strokes. Consider opening out your fingers for 10 strokes, allowing your arms to move freely to help diffuse some fatigue and then continue.

Bike techniques—Stretch a little by getting out of the saddle on a flat section of road, open up your lungs, take in some deep breaths, then resume cycling. Do this every 20 minutes. Spin an easier gear when it's time to change to a gear with more resistance and after the crest of a hill, wait 5 seconds to allow your muscles to recover.

Focusing too far into the distance or how far you have to go is likely to stop you from thinking about your hydration and nutrition.

Run techniques—Drop your arms and shake out, relax loose fingers, let your shoulders drop, release tension. All this is good to do when you are feeling tense and tired. Then bring your arms back to 45 degrees and continue to run.

OVERCOME INDIVIDUAL FEARS

Overcome the fears in your mind then link them up into one image before filing them away. Brush aside any insecurity that may happen at any time.

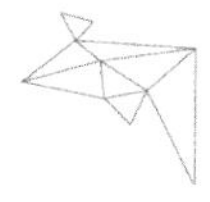

"Trust yourself, you know more than you think you do."
Benjamin Spock

Problem-solving strategies should be segmented and linked together when considering how you are feeling, comparing your personal performance, coping with the environment, and comparing yourself with others.

Self-talk is not about confrontation; it is about your positive thoughts overcoming your negative thoughts.

Make the positive crowd of voices in your head larger for "I can do this," "I have trained in harder conditions" or "I have come a long way to get here," or simply have your own mental key to unlock these positive thoughts. You will soon experience the negative thoughts being drowned by your mind for a mental victory.

Think of the elation you will experience crossing the finish line.

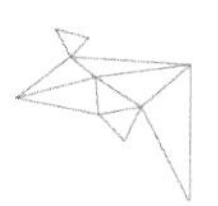

"Do not dwell in the past, do not dream of the future, concentrate the mind on the present moment." Buddha

AVOIDANCE STRATEGY

This can be equally successful and is also known as dissociation. Thinking about something else during your triathlon.

For example, think of doing all the things you have not been able to do while preparing for your triathlon.

But a word of warning that these thoughts should not put you in a trance-like mental state so that you are unaware of what is going on around you.

Generally, the more experienced a triathlete you are the fewer concerns you will have unless you failed to address problems in the past with a potential coping strategy. Work on any issues that might cause you anxiety by creating mental imagery now, not during race week.

A large number of experienced triathletes worry about things within their control simply because they have not devoted time to thinking of a fear or going through what they would do if it happened.

So how can a first-timer or someone with less experience overcome adversity? Simply by generating as much mental imagery as possible, thinking about race week, controlling your nerves before arriving at the triathlon, registration, transition, putting on your wetsuit, and getting to the swim start.

The more times you have thought through possible situations and overcome them in your mind, like a world-class chess player, it is much easier it will be to make the right decision while relaxed and on autopilot.

Many first-time or experienced triathletes I have advised experience less stress on triathlon day simply because they have gone through all the possible worst-case scenarios in their minds.

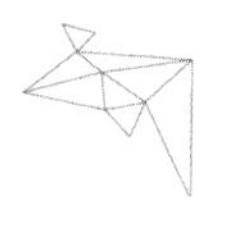

"What would life be if we had no courage to attempt anything?"

Vincent van Gogh

10.2 SUMMARY: HOW TO BE A BETTER PERSON AND ATHLETE BY TAKING CONTROL OF YOUR MIND

MISTAKES TO AVOID

Instant replay mental rehearsal is the most common but most hit-and-miss method used. The triathlete only goes over the triathlon in their mind just before or just afterward. This is often counter-productive. A gymnast will take as long as the routine and a Formula One driver or MotoGP rider will take as long as a lap. They will also go into more detail about warm-up laps and racing scenarios plus media obligations just before competing.

In triathlon, it is simply not possible to spend the same amount of time mentally rehearsing as the swim-bike-run is going to take you.

Think about small, bite-sized parts of the race and join these parts up in the many weeks before the triathlon. Occassionally fast forward the complete image from start to finish. If you can't do this seamlessly, go back to areas in your mind where the imagery seems to be a problem and make another personal thought of what you hope to achieve.

Our bodies and minds have an amazing ability to remember what we have done before. Use imagery to kickstart your event and make yourself better.

Creative distraction is helpful when you find it hard to keep positive. Thanking a marshal or smiling at the spectators will greatly help.

Every human being makes errors and if we repeat these errors, they become mistakes. Think of a mistake as a learning opportunity and use this experience for the future.

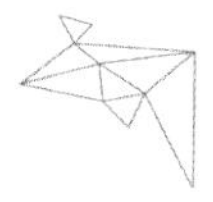

"Plans are only good intentions, start your good intentions today starting with mental imagery." Mark Kleanthous

10.3 COPING STRATEGIES: SELECTION AND EFFECTIVENESS IN RELATION TO ANTICIPATED AND ACUTE RACE STRESSORS ENCOUNTERED BY NON-ELITE LONG-DISTANCE MALE TRIATHLETES

By Mr. Peter Hayward

This study was kindly provided by Peter Hayward who achieved a degree (first-class honors) and gained an A for his dissertation in the above study. A part of this dissertation has been included in this book.

The following study confirms my own personal experience coaching athletes and my investigations asking hundreds of triathletes about effective coping strategies in triathlon.

This study involved long distance age group triathletes

FAST FACTS

Age range–35 to 59 years (mean = 48 years)

Triathlon Experience–between 1 and 37 Ironman® events (mean average 8.4 long distance triathlon events per triathlete involved in the study)

The study was conducted in 3 main stages

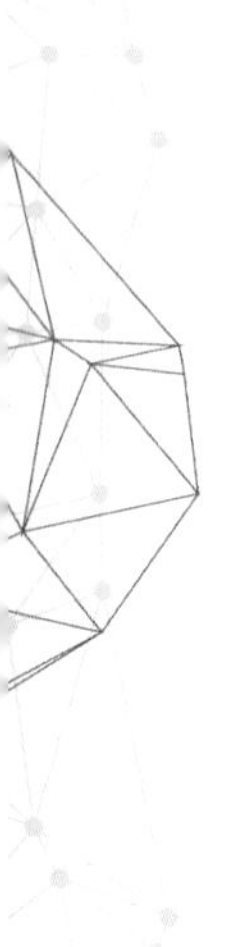

1. Standardized pre-race open-ended questionnaire
2. Post-race prompt questionnaire including rate of perceived control over stress on a 4-point scale.
3. List of stressors questionnaire completed within 12 hours of finishing the triathlon. Open-ended prompts: "Please list the stressors you encountered during your race in order of highest to lowest distress, both expected and unexpected;" and "For each of the stressors you listed please indicate and describe any coping strategies you applied. If they felt no coping strategy was used they indicated 'none.'" Give a

point of 0 to 4 to the effectiveness of coping strategy they employed from "totally to not at all" (a "not applicable" option was available if no coping strategy was used).

The aim of this study was to examine the effectiveness of coping strategies employed by non-elite long-distance male triathletes in response to anticipated and acute race stressors. The findings of the study reveal that the most frequently reported anticipated race stressors were mechanical/equipment failure, injury, environmental factors and the swim start of the race. However, the most saliently reported acute race stressors were injury, environmental factors, the other athletes and the race course. It is important to recognize that these particular stressors are specific to long-distance triathlon as reported by the triathletes questioned but appear to be common stressors to the majority of triathletes.

The tables below are a summary of the study on endurance triathletes and reflect an overview of the range of performance-related stressors and coping strategies themes rather than describe them all individually in detail.

Table 4.1. An overview of the number of athletes reporting particular stressors and the total number of citations reported. Results are derived from the deductive data analysis.

	Anticipated		Acute In-race	
Stressors	No. of Athletes (n = 7)	No. of Citations	No. of Athletes (n = 7)	No. of Citations
Mechanical/equipment failure	6	7	2	3
Injury	5	6	7	11
Environmental factors	5	6	7	11
Swim start	4	4	3	3
Nutrition/hydration	4	4	1	1
Race course/Organization	4	4	4	7
Exhaustion	3	3	2	3
Illness	2	4	2	2
Performance	2	2	3	3
Other athletes	2	2	5	6
Biological needs	2	2	1	1
Natural world	0	0	2	3
Nerves	0	0	1	1

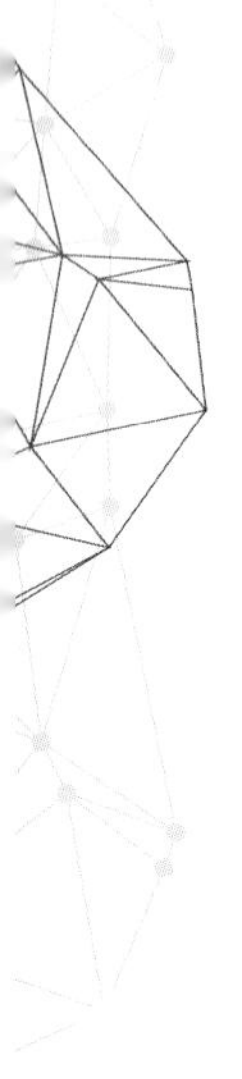

Table 4.2. An overview of the number of athletes reporting each coping strategy dimension and the total number of citations for each. Results are derived from the deductive data analysis.

	Pre-race		Acute In-race	
Coping Strategies	No. of Athletes (n = 7)	No. of Citations	No. of Athletes (n = 7)	No. of Citations
Problem-focused (total)	7	55	7	38
Physical preparation	7	17	0	0
Controlling effort	5	9	7	11
Planning	4	11	4	4
Strategy orientated	3	6	4	4
Problem solving	2	6	6	7
Mental preparation	2	2	0	0
Physical Avoidance	2	2	5	6
Information Seeking	1	2	0	0
Change behavior	1	1	2	2
Nutrition orientated	0	0	3	4
Emotion-focused (total)	6	22	7	55
Re-appraisal	4	4	4	4
Positive orientation	2	4	3	3
Experience/Self-confidence	2	4	4	6
Social support	2	3	5	7
Positive self-talk	2	2	7	13
Acceptance	1	3	3	6
Rationalizing	1	1	2	2
Relaxation/Visualization	1	1	4	4
Wishful thinking	0	0	3	4
Humor	0	0	2	4

	Pre-race		Acute In-race	
Venting emotions	0	0	2	2
Avoidance				
(total)	4	5	5	9
Lack of strategy	3	4	2	2
Thought stopping	1	1	0	0
Cognitive avoidance	0	0	3	4
Distraction	0	0	2	2
Drugs	0	0	1	1

The above provides in detail the most frequently reported anticipated stressors the athlete felt they had and the coping strategies utilized to minimize the anxiety. The most frequently reported anticipated stressors were mechanical/equipment failure, injury, environmental factors, the swim start and nutrition/hydration (Table 4.1). In coping with these stressors, the athletes predominantly reported problem-focused coping strategies, of which physical preparation, controlling effort and planning were most cited (Table 4.2).

It is therefore recommended that athletes incorporate mental skills development into their training programs.

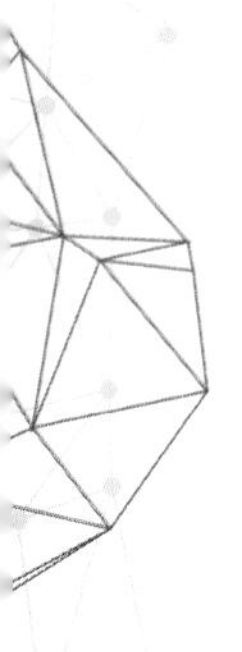

10.3.1 EXAMPLE TRIATHLETE FEARS & EFFECTIVE COPING STRATEGIES:

There are various kinds of stressors that an athlete can encounter during a long-distance triathlon. These stressors can include physical such as injury, cramping and exhaustion, external environmental such as equipment failure and adverse weather conditions, and psychological and emotional such as low self-esteem or self-confidence.

Please list all the stressors you could expect to encounter during the race in order of highest to lowest concern (please continue overleaf if you need more space).

STRESSOR

1. The fear of drowning during the triathlon swim.
2. I dehydrated, got cramps and was not able to finish my triathlon.
3. Mechanical bike failure. I was concerned that if I had a problem with my bike I would not be able to finish the cycle section of the triathlon and not finish.
4. I was worried about not being able to get to swim in a straight line which would mean banging into others and losing time during the triathlon.
5. The Swim start–Getting kicked in the face.
6. I was worried I would be nervous which would affect me thinking clearly.
7. I was worried I would get a flat tyre and not be able to change it or lose valuable time during the triathlon.
8. I was worried about getting blisters from not wearing socks to save time in transition between swim and bike.

Please indicate the appropriate level of **control** you feel you have over each stressor, according to the specific stressors you listed above, on the scale below.

Stressor 1:	Full	Full to Medium	Some	Minimal	None
Stressor 2:	Full	Full to Medium	Some	Minimal	None
Stressor 3:	Full	Full to Medium	Some	Minimal	None
Stressor 4:	Full	Full to Medium	Some	Minimal	None
Stressor 5:	Full	Full to Medium	Some	Minimal	None
Stressor 6:	Full	Full to Medium	Some	Minimal	None
Stressor 7:	Full	Full to Medium	Some	Minimal	None
Stressor 8:	Full	Full to Medium	Some	Minimal	None

AWARD THE FOLLOWING POINTS:

- **Full = 5 points**

  Very stressful and you feel you are not in complete control.

- **Full to Medium = 4 points**

  This feels like waves that increase from medium to full fear then ease slightly. The slightest thing can increase anxiety.

- **Some = 3 points**

  This is healthy fear. Allows you to be "Race Ready", in control and ready to compete. You should be able to think clearly under pressure with some fear.

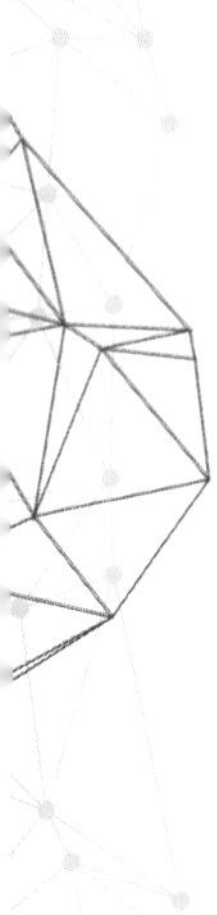

- **Minimal = 2 points**

  You have naturally considered this a low level anxiety. Low fear or arousal can actually be counterproductive to being completely race ready.

- **None = 0 points**

  You have mentally rehearsed your fears and they no longer concern you because you can deal with them. If and when they occur you can go into automatic pilot without any worries.

For each of the stressors you listed above please indicate any coping strategies you may have put in place.

They can be listed in order of priority or any order. It is important to give them your realistic fear you have.

1. I practised floating in my wet suit and tried to dive down and experienced it was impossible to sink and drown.
2. I set my watch to bleep every 10 minutes during the bike and run to remind me to hydrate in training. Eventually, I drank without needing my stop watch to bleep. I never experienced cramps in training or in my triathlon.
3. I booked my bike into the local bike shop 3 weeks before and got the brake and gear cables changed and they checked the bike. This gave me the confidence during my final taper and on triathlon race day.
4. I learnt to swim in a straight line by looking up and sighting every two strokes, then every four, then every six, then eight strokes. During the triathlon, I glanced every four strokes and monitored landmarks ahead and to my side to keep me swimming in a straight line.
5. I practise fast swim starts in training with friends who were slower and faster than me. This gave me confidence that although we were swimming in close proximity in training my face or goggles never got knocked off.
6. I thought about every part of the triathlon, what could go wrong and how I could overcome it and I felt far more relaxed and less nervous than I thought I would be. This has given me even more confidence for future triathlons.
7. By changing the tyre many times I was able to get back on the road in a couple of minutes. During this time I chewed on a sports bar so I could easily absorb it while fixing the flat so once back on the road I could make up some time cycling.

For extra peace of mind I replaced my tyres with new ones two weeks before my triathlon and checked them the day before and on race day for any cuts or flints etc.

8. I trained without wearing socks and used a small amount of Vaseline in my shoes as extra protective. I never got blisters so will not worry in the future.

Please rate how **effective** you felt the coping strategy was in reducing the distress the stressor caused on the scale below.

Stressor 1:	Totally	Mostly	Little	Not at all	N/A
Stressor 2:	Totally	Mostly	Little	Not at all	N/A
Stressor 3:	Totally	Mostly	Little	Not at all	N/A
Stressor 4:	Totally	Mostly	Little	Not at all	N/A
Stressor 5:	Totally	Mostly	Little	Not at all	N/A
Stressor 6:	Totally	Mostly	Little	Not at all	N/A
Stressor 7:	Totally	Mostly	Little	Not at all	N/A
Stressor 8:	Totally	Mostly	Little	Not at all	N/A

AWARD THE FOLLOWING POINTS:

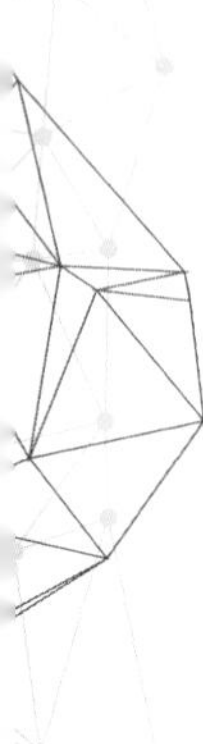

- **Totally = 4 points**
  You completely overcome your fears
- **Mostly = 3 points**
  You overcome your fears
- **Little = 2 points**
  You hardly reduced your fear levels
- **Not at all = 1 point**
  It made no difference

- **N/A = award yourself the same number as you gave it before the triathlon**
  This situation did not happen to you.

SUMMARY OF EXAMPLE TRIATHLETE

An example triathlete reduced their pre triathlon score from 33 points before the triathlon by 11 points by effectively using effective coping strategies.

If you can reduce the number of points you have scored from 4 weeks before your triathlon to race week then you have effectively used practise and mental imagery to help you.

If you have reduced the number of points you scored the week before to after your triathlon then you have used your experience to good use.

Recall these reduced levels of fears for the future training and triathlon competitions.

Use the blank form below pre and post triathlon.

The above table was kindly provided by Peter Hayward who achieved a First Class honours degree Sports science.

10.3.2 COPING STRATEGIES: SELECTION AND EFFECTIVENESS TRIATHLETES

PERSONAL INFORMATION

Name:

a) Please list the stressors you encountered during your race in order of highest to lowest distress, both expected and unexpected (please use more examples if you need to.

1.

2.

3.

4.

5.

6.

7.

8.

b) Please indicate the appropriate level of control you feel you had over each stressor during the race, according to the specific stressors you listed above, on the scale below.

Stressor 1:	100%	75%	50%	less than 25%	Not at all
Stressor 2:	100%	75%	50%	less than 25%	Not at all
Stressor 3:	100%	75%	50%	less than 25%	Not at all
Stressor 4:	100%	75%	50%	less than 25%	Not at all
Stressor 5:	100%	75%	50%	less than 25%	Not at all
Stressor 6:	100%	75%	50%	less than 25%	Not at all
Stressor 7:	100%	75%	50%	less than 25%	Not at all
Stressor 8:	100%	75%	50%	less than 25%	Not at all

c) For each of the stressors you listed above please indicate and describe any coping strategies you applied. If you feel no coping strategy was used please indicate 'none'.

1. ______________________________

2. ______________________________

3. ______________________________

4. ______________________________

5. ______________________________

6. ______________________________

7. ______________________________

8. ______________________________

d) Please rate how effective you felt the coping strategy was in reducing the distress the stressor caused on the scale below.

Stressor 1:	Totally	Mostly	Little	Not at all	N/A
Stressor 1:	Totally	Mostly	Little	Not at all	N/A
Stressor 1:	Totally	Mostly	Little	Not at all	N/A
Stressor 1:	Totally	Mostly	Little	Not at all	N/A
Stressor 1:	Totally	Mostly	Little	Not at all	N/A
Stressor 1:	Totally	Mostly	Little	Not at all	N/A
Stressor 1:	Totally	Mostly	Little	Not at all	N/A
Stressor 1:	Totally	Mostly	Little	Not at all	N/A

Points scoring system for above:

- **Totally = 4 points**
  You completely overcome your fears.
- **Mostly = 3 points**
  You overcome your fears.
- **Little = 2 points**
  You hardly reduced your fear levels.
- **Not a all = 1 point**
  It made no difference.
- **N/A = award yourself same number as you gave yourself before the triathlon**
  This situation did not happen to you.

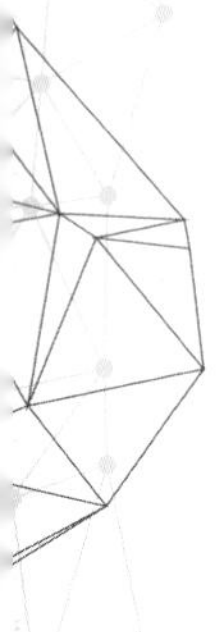

The purpose is to reduce the number of points post-race. The bigger the percentage reduction, the greater the gains. A triathlete who reduces their score from 32 to 24 shows a reduction of 25% which is similar to a triathlete who originally scored 20 and reduced their score to 15 points.

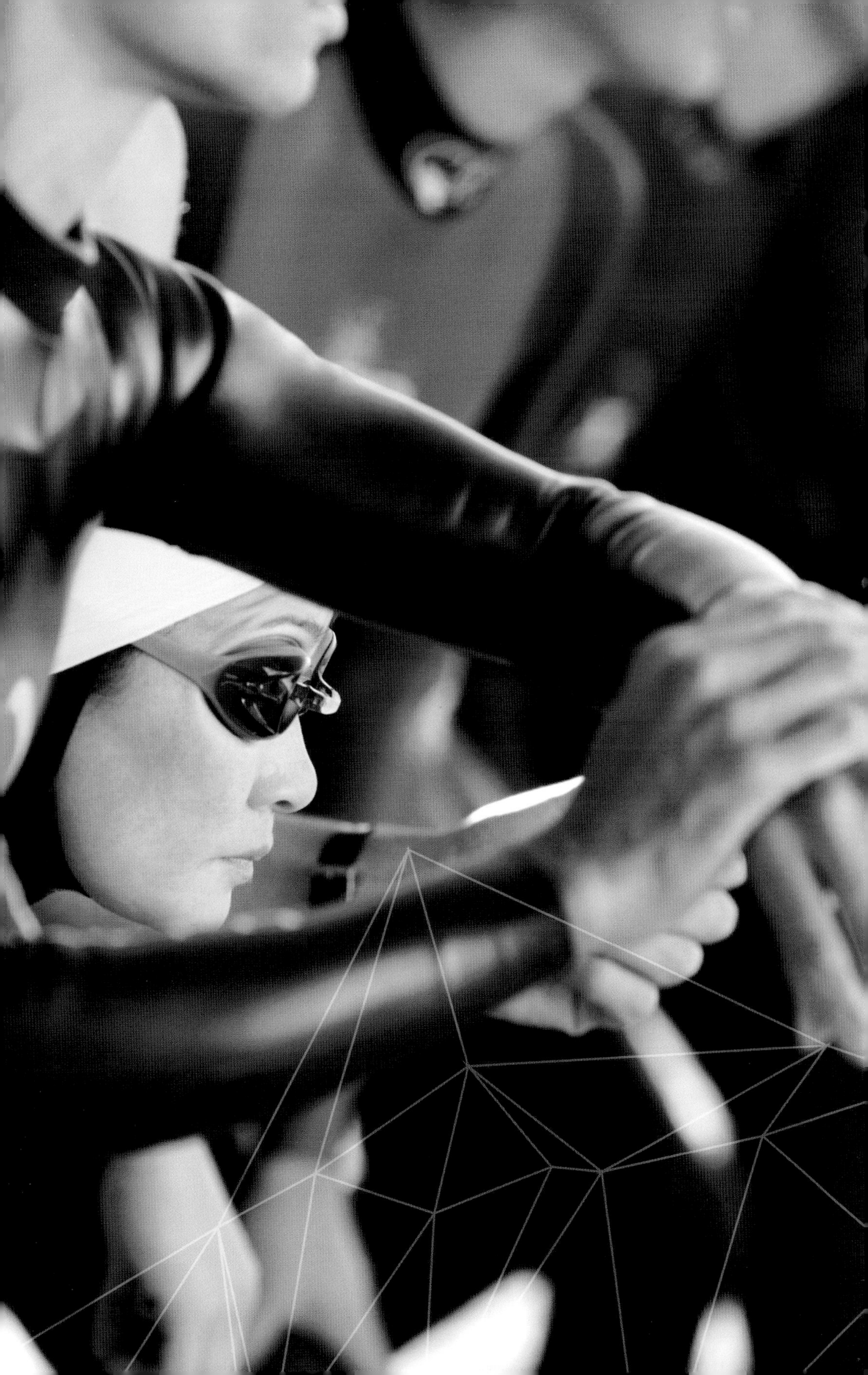

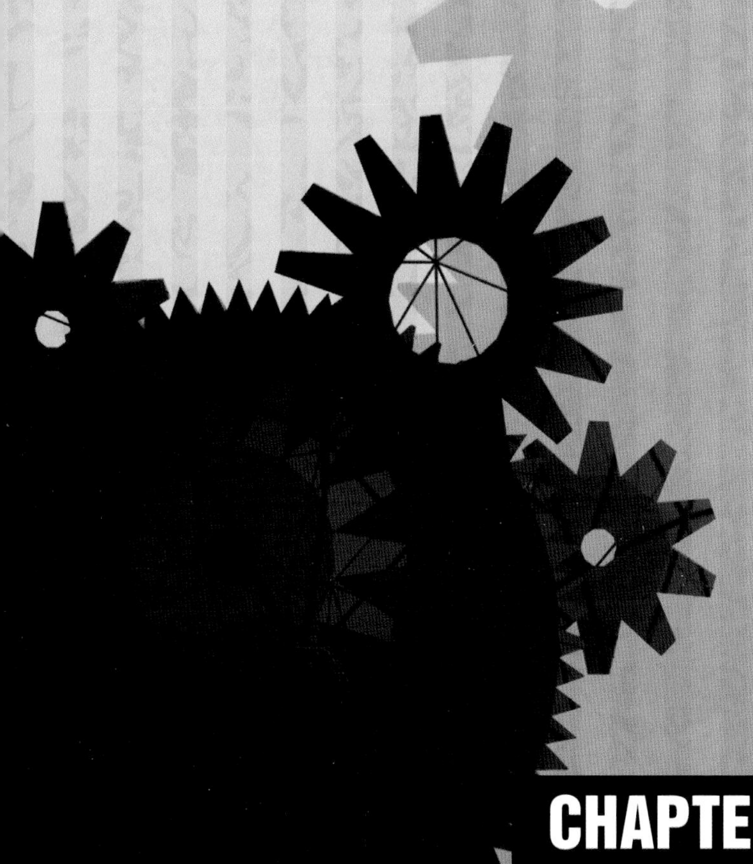

CHAPTER ELEVEN.

TAKE AWAY TIPS FROM THIS BOOK

ELEVEN.

TAKE AWAY TIPS FROM THIS BOOK

- Recognize cause for anxiety and aim to reduce it to a manageable level.
- Mentally rehearse looking at yourself and imagining yourself in the triathlon.
- Aim to get to a mindset where you have effortless concentration.
- Don't just act the race, feel the triathlon and try and experience the emotions. An actress will not just read her lines, she will add expression and movement.
- Watch yourself looking from the inside and from the outside.
- Find a quiet place and time early in the morning before the pace of the day builds up.
- Practice at a similar time of day, ideally when you will be competing in your triathlon.
- Think about obstacles that may happen and how you are going to overcome them—never just act out a perfect triathlon.
- If you are tense before the start of your triathlon, remember that tensions are released with movement, so once you start you will be fine.
- Associate thinking about the here and now during the triathlon and don't forget any part of what you have practiced.
- To dissociate is to daydream. When things get tough on race day, use it as a distraction.
- Ignore non-essential distractions.
- Don't confuse the sensation of fear with excitement.
- Do not ignore your fears, but do not spend considerable time on your fears either.

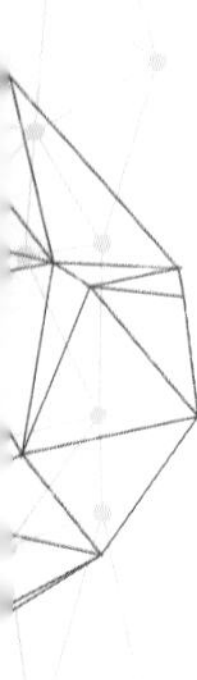

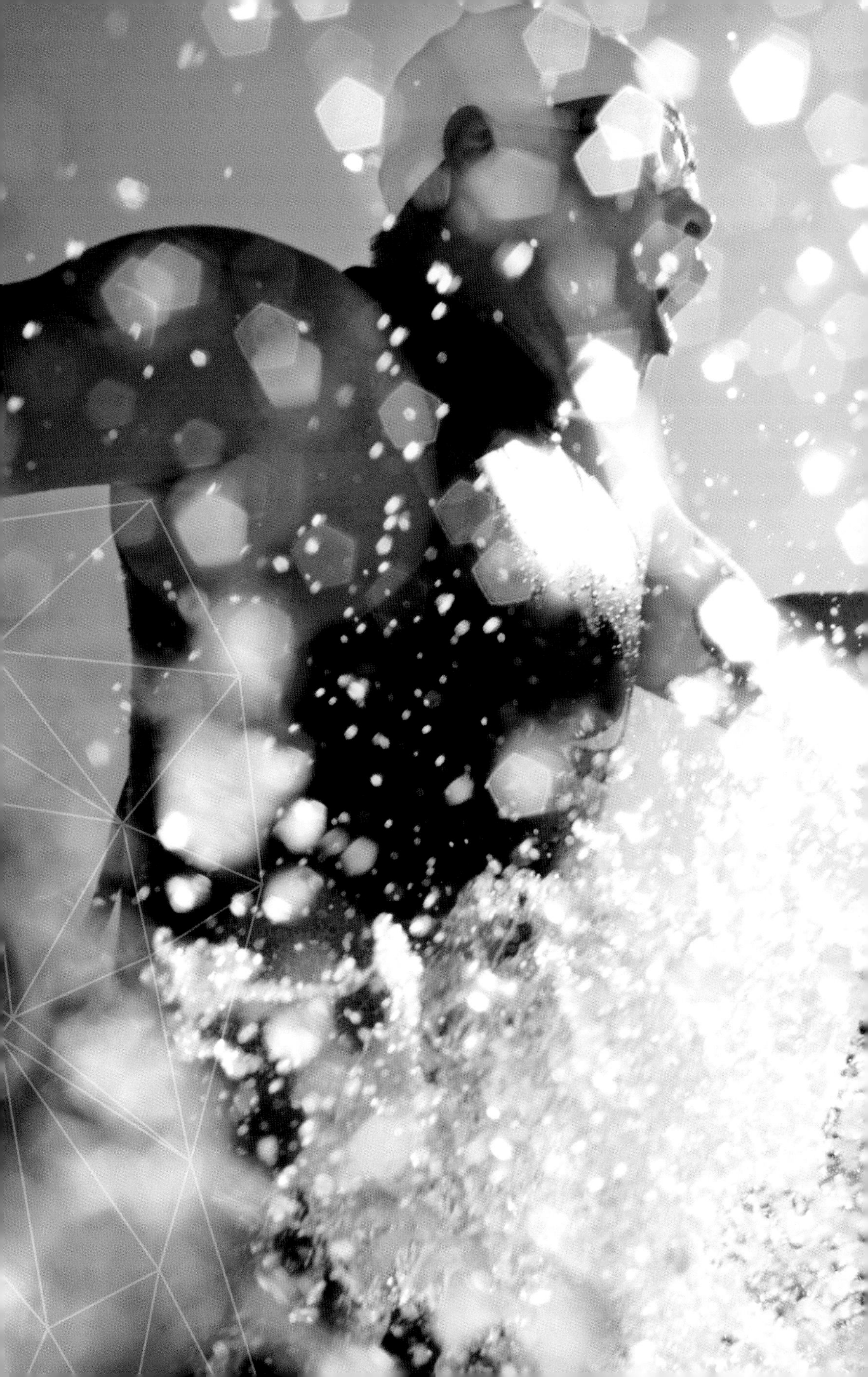

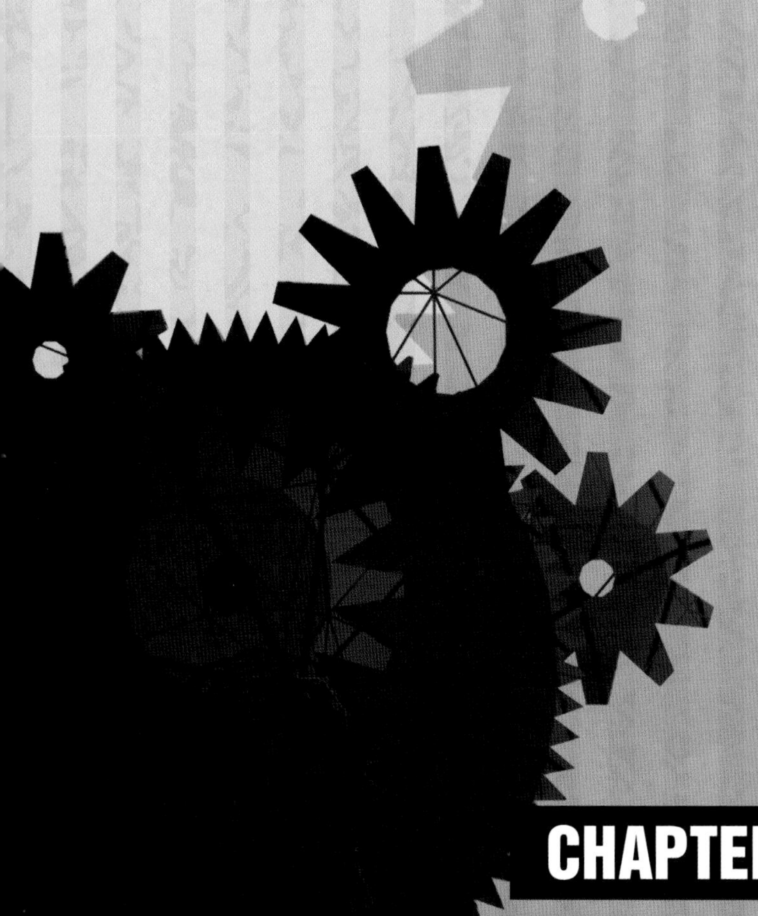

CHAPTER TWELVE.

A TO Z OF THE SPORTING MIND

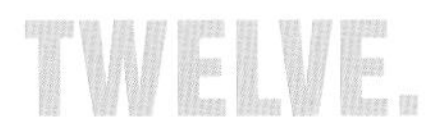

TWELVE.
A TO Z OF THE SPORTING MIND

Words associated with the sporting mind	
Adrenaline	Hormone secreted by the adrenal medulla upon stimulation by the central nervous system
Aggressive mind	Unjustly attacking mentally or physically
Analytical thinking	Reasoning or acting from a perception of parts andinterrelations of a subject
Angry	Feeling or showing anger; incensed or enraged
Anxiety	State of uneasiness and apprehension, as about future uncertainties
Assertive	Between being passive and aggressive. If passive, you do not vocalize your thoughts; if aggressive, you have frustrations. Assertive is confident and self-assured
Attitude	A state of mind or a feeling; disposition
Attunement	To adjust or accustom; acclimatize
Autopilot thinking	Doing something without thinking about what you are doing, usually because you have done it many times before
Balanced judgment	The power or means to decide
Bargaining mind	To arrive at an agreement
Body language	Gestures, postures, and facial expressions by which a person manifests various physical, mental or emotional states
Brainstorming	A method of shared problem solving in which all members of a group simultaneously contribute ideas
Breathing techniques	Using breathing to relax (see chapter on physical rehearsal techniques)
Chattering mind	To think rapidly, incessantly and often on trivial subjects

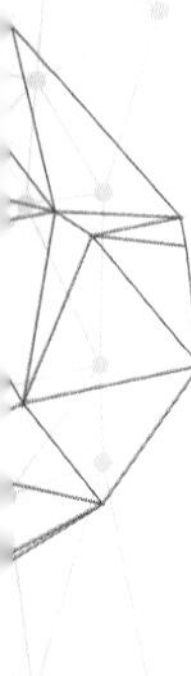

Words associated with the sporting mind	
Chill	A cool, calm, collected relaxed mental state of mind that helps the body to also be relaxed
Choking	A feeling you're suffocating or cannot breathe; the feeling you're failing or doing poorly when the advantages were there to win
Competitive mindset	Of, involving or determined by competition
Composure	A calm or tranquil state of mind; self-possession
Concentration, good	Act or process of concentrating, especially the fixing of close, undivided attention
Concentration, loss of	Unable to concentrate sufficiently
Confidence	Trust or faith in a person or thing; feeling of self-assurance
Conscience	Awareness of moral or ethical aspect of one's conduct with an urge to prefer right over wrong
Constructive criticism	Positive and negative opinion offered in a friendly manner
Decision-making	The cognitive process of reaching a decision
Defeatism	A ready acceptance or expectation of defeat
Denial	A refusal to grant the truth of a statement or allegation
Destructive	Something that is disproving, discrediting or negative
Dichotomous thinking	Divided or dividing into two parts or classifications
Dislikes	Signifies a need to change your attitude. One example could be "I don't like cold water but my wetsuit will help keep me warm"
Distractions	Something that serves as a diversion, possibly mental or emotional
Doubts	To be undecided or sceptical about various things
Dysfunction	Abnormal or impaired functioning especially of a bodily system

Words associated with the sporting mind	
Effective coping strategies	Contend or strive, especially on even terms or with success
Ego	The self, especially as distinct from the world and other selves
Emotional thinking	Readily affected with or stirred by emotion
Enthusiasm	Great excitement for or interest in a subject or cause
Eventuality thinking	Forward thoughts of an event, occurrence or result
Excitement	Stimulation or thrill of various events
Expectations, realistic, unrealistic	Eager anticipation, something anticipated, not compatible with reality or fact, unreasonably idealistic
Failure	Feeling of not achieving the desired goal or proper performance
Fear	Feeling of agitation and anxiety possibly caused by presence of danger
Fight	Attempt to gain power over an adversary by striving vigorously and resolutely
Flight	Rapid movement or progress
Freeze	Feeling of agitation and immobilization with fear or shock
Goal setting	The purpose toward an endeavor is directed as an objective
Hijacking mind	Good thoughts overshadowed by bad thoughts
Home advantage	Competing on a course where you live or train regularly. Can give the triathlete a psychological advantage and improve confidence levels
Hostile crowds	Unfriendly onlookers
Indecision	Reluctance or an inability to make up one's mind
Inner mind	The link between the spirit and the body, often referred to as imagination
Instant replay	Recording and immediate playback of a sporting event
Intimidation	To coerce, inhibit or frighten into submission
Intonation	Manner of producing or uttering tones with regard to accuracy

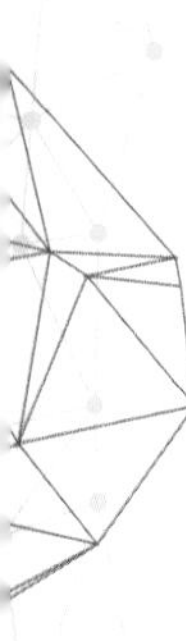

Words associated with the sporting mind	
Jitters	To be nervous or uneasy
Journal technique	Writing down your thoughts will slow down your thinking mind and help with "what's on your mind." Don't worry about grammar, neatness, spelling, or clarity. You have to slow down thinking automatically because you cannot write as quick as you can speak
Kinesthetic inventory	Sense that detects bodily position, weight or movement of the muscles, tendons and joints
Logical thinking	Process of using your mind to consider something carefully
Malfunction	An event that does not accomplish its intended purpose
Malleability	The brain's ability or reorganizing itself if it is damaged by an accident or stroke and can have the ability to take over functions of another part of the brain
Mantra	Sacred verbal formula repeated in prayer, meditation or incantation. Many triathletes have their own and often their partners do not even know them
Medication	Something that treats or prevents symptoms of disease
Mental evaluation	This is the equivalent of a physical examination. During a competition, the mind should be self-checking itself for signs of fatigue, thirst, energy levels and any muscle tightness
Mental rehearsal techniques	A great way to improve skill, behavior, reflex actions, overcoming adversity, and athletic performance. t is also known as "imagined practice" and can reduce stress and boost confidence and help you make the correct decision if things do not go as planned.
Mental toughness	Hard to define–words used to describe include self-sacrifice, resilience, focus, preparation, handling pressure, motivation self-belief, inner desire, determination
Mentally disconnect	Close your eyes breathe deeply and focus on a great performance that you have mentally rehearsed time and time again

Words associated with the sporting mind	
Mind games	Calculate psychological thoughts to make you mentally and physically stronger. Can also be used to cause confusion intimidate for a competitive advantage
Motivation	That which can be defended by reasoning or logical argument
Negative criticism	Lacking positive or affirmative qualities
Nerves	Nervousness resulting from mental stress
Overacting	To act over and above what is required
Painting a picture	Mental image of something, like a racecourse
Paranoid	Exhibiting extreme and irrational fear or distrust of others
Performance review	Analyzing one's performance
Personality types	Sporting personality types: **Introverts** tend to enjoy sports that require the following skills: Concentration, individual performances, intricate details, low or constant arousal levels, precision, self-motivation. Partial aggression can be used to dig deep and try and beat another triathlete in a completion **Extroverts** tend to enjoy sports that require the following skills: Exciting, high arousal levels, team sports, fast paces, low concentration levels, power sports, football, rugby and motorsports attract this type of individual. Indirect aggression taking aggression and stress out on an object like a punching bag, tennis ball, golf ball, football. Direct aggression personality types take aggression out on another player with direct contact like in boxing, rugby, wrestling, judo, etc. Every person is different and some people have traits from each type.
Positive self-imagery	Conception that one has of oneself regarding qualities and personal worth
Pressure	An oppressive condition of physical and mental distress
Prioritize	Assign a priority to what you want to achieve
Proactive	Acting in advance to deal with an expected difficulty

Words associated with the sporting mind	
Psyched	To put into the right psychological frame of mind
Psychoanalysis	This transfers from the past to present. This can be the fear of water from childhood brought to a current situation. Known as the deep-seated unconscious template of life. This can result in unconscious conflict causing fear nerves, etc.
Psychological evaluations	Jobs or courts may require psychological assessments, so as a triathlete you should also look at your mental state of mind
Quiet place	Quiet place to clear your mind can be lying still, closing your eyes in a quiet place like the library, a walk in the woods with no distractions, turn off your phone, think of a relaxing situation, arrange some flowers, sit and watch the river go by or look out into a lake and watch the ripples. My favorite was a walk in the giant redwoods forests.
Rage	A feeling of intense anger
Reflection	Continuous and profound contemplation of previous events
Regret	Feeling of disappointment or distress about something that could be different
Relaxation techniques	These include breathing, humming, meditation, getting in tune with your senses, and journal techniques
Responsive reaction	
Self-control	Control of one's emotions, desires or actions by one's own will
Self-confidence	Self-assuredness in one's personal judgment and ability
Self-esteem	A feeling of self-respect and personal worth
Self-image	The conception that one has of oneself including qualities and personal worth
Self-worth	Self-worth is an essential human need that is vital for survival, get up and go, and is normal for a healthy existence. Self-esteem can be self-worth, self-respect, or self-value

Words associated with the sporting mind	
Stress, chronic and healthy stress	Chronic stress can wreak havoc on your mind and body. Healthy stress is a natural way to protect you from predators and aggression. For the majority of people in peaceful times, thankfully this is rare. A dog barking is stressful until you establish it is on a chain and behind a closed gate. Make sure you reduce your stress. Stress in modern life comes from commuting to work deadlines, problems with your computer, earning enough to pay your bills, etc. Controlling your stress is healthy.
Stress, types of	**Acute stress** does not cause long-term health issues associated with long-term stress. It usually happens to people who are always in a rush, do not plan and always leave late. **Emotional distress** can be one of the following or a combination of anger, depression, irritability, muscular tension, headaches, or stomach pain, heartburn, back pain, muscle aches and pains. **Episode stress** is on-going stress; the smallest of things cause you stress. **Chronic stress** is experienced by those who cannot see a way out of a miserable or difficult situation. The pressure seems unbearable.
Tension	Mental, emotional or nervous strain
Traumatic memory	Recollection of serious injury or shock to the system
Unfinished business	Activity directed towards making or doing something that's incomplete
Unrealistic goals or expectations	Goals that one makes that are beyond their ability at the current time, such as expecting to win an Ironman® on your first go
Values	Beliefs of a person in which they have an emotional investment
Visualization	An iconic mental representation similar to a visual perception

Words associated with the sporting mind	
Will power	The strength of will to carry out one's decisions, wishes or plans
Worrying	Feeling uneasy or concerned about something
Yearning	Persistent, often wistful desire or longing
Zone mode	Narrow, focused mind and believing in your current fitness levels and ability

CHAPTER THIRTEEN.

A TO Z OF NEGATIVE WORDS

THIRTEEN.

A TO Z OF NEGATIVE WORDS

It's important to change negative thoughts to positive thoughts! Choose a different word that means less negativity to you!

A to Z of negative words:	Meaning:
Adverse	Harmful or negative
Afraid	Frightened or apprehensive
Alarming	Disturbing or intimidating
Angry	Annoyed or furious
Annoy	Irritate or hassle
Anxious	Expectant or uneasy
Apathy	Emotionless or indifference
Appalling	Frightening or distressing
Atrocious	Detestable or terrible
Awful	Unpleasant or nauseous
Bad	Unfavorable or damaging
Beneath	Under or unworthy
Blisters	Cysts or carbuncles
Boring	Tedious or uninteresting
Broken	Injured or damaged
Can't	Cannot or unable
Cheating	Deception or unfaithful
Clumsy	Awkward or uncoordinated
Cold	Unloving or chilliness
Cold-hearted	Insensitive or heartless
Collapse	Breakdown or blackout
Confused	Bewildered or perplexed
Contradictory	Inconsistent or conflicting
Contrary	Differing or opposing

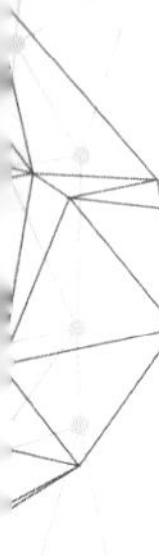

A to Z of negative words:	Meaning:
Crazy	Ridiculous or eccentric
Cruel	Ruthless or remorseless
Cry	Weep or tearful
Damaging	Harmful or detrimental
DNF	Did not finish
DNS	Did not start
Deny	Refute or repudiate
Depressed	Despondent or pessimistic
Deprived	Disadvantaged or underprivileged
Despicable	Contemptible or reprehensible
Detrimental	Unfavorable or damaging
Disease	Illness or affliction
Disgusting	Sickening or distasteful
Dismal	Dreadful or depressing
Distress	Anguish or anxiety
Don't	Stop or curtail
Doubts	Uncertainty or skepticism
Dreadful	Distressing or appalling
Dreary	Monotonous or tedious
Exhausted	Drained or fatigued
Fail	Unsuccessful or disappointed
Faulty	Imperfect or malfunctioning
Fear	Consternation or fright
Feeble	Exhausted or delicate
Fight	Withstand or overcome
Filthy	Squalid or unclean
Frighten	Terrorize or scare
Frightful	Horrifying or atrocious
Gawky	Ungainly or graceless
Ghastly	Shocking or dreadful
Grave	Serious or threatening

A to Z of negative words:	Meaning:
Greed	Insatiable or craving
Grim	Depressing or forbidding
Grimace	Scowl or wince
Gross	Horrible or large
Grotesque	Ludicrous or strange
Gruesome	Shocking or hideous
Guilty	Responsible or ashamed
Haggard	Gaunt or emaciated
Hard	Tough or exhausting
Hard-hearted	Unsympathetic or insensitive
Harmful	Damaging or unhealthy
Hate	Despise or detest
Hideous	Ghastly or gruesome
Hilly	Undulating or rough
Homely	Comfortable or welcoming
Horrendous	Appalling or fearsome
Horrible	Dreadful or unpleasant
Hot	Humid or sweltering
Hurt	Injured or wounded
Hurtful	Unkind or harmful
Ignore	Disregard or overlook
Illness	Malaise or ailment
Immature	Childish or undeveloped
Imperfect	Flawed or defective
Impossible	Impracticable or unachievable
Injure	Wound or damage
Insane	Irrational or deranged
Insidious	Cunning or subtle
Jealous	Possessive or apprehensive
Lose	Forfeit or outrun
Lousy	Terrible or inferior

A to Z of negative words:	Meaning:
Malicious	Spiteful or malevolent
Mean	Miserly or malicious
Menacing	Threatening or intimidating
Misshapen	Deformed or unshapely
Missing	Absent or nonexistent
Misunderstood	Misconstrued or misunderstood
Moan	Complain or grumble
Monstrous	Outrageous or atrocious
Naïve	Gullible or inexperienced
Nasty	Unpleasant or distasteful
Negative	Pessimistic or unsupportive
Nervous	Tense or agitated
Never	Giving up, giving in
No	Opposite to yes
Nobody	No-one or nonentity
Nonsense	Rubbish or stupidity
Not	Emotional feeling stronger than no
Noxious	Harmful or unhealthy
Objectionable	Unacceptable or offensive
Old	Elderly or outmoded
Oppressive	Overwhelming or domineering
Pain	Discomfort or distress
Panic	Anxiety or consternation
Pessimistic	Foreboding or despairing
Petty	Insignificant or unimportant
Plain	Simple or Spartan
Poor	Impoverished or unfortunate
Problems	Difficulties or obstacles
Questionable	Dubious or uncertain
Quirky	Unconventional or offbeat
Quit	Discontinue or withdraw

A to Z of negative words:	Meaning:
Reject	Abandon or relinquish
Repulsive	Offensive or abhorrent
Revenge	Retaliation or retribution
Revolting	Disgusting or nauseating
Rocky	Unstable or rough
Rotten	Disintegrating or festering
Sad	Unhappy or depressed
Savage	Harsh or ruthless
Scare	Frighten or intimidate
Scary	Alarming or chilling
Scream	Shriek or screech
Severe	Serious or intense
Shocking	Appalling or horrendous
Sick	Unwell or poorly
Sickening	Disgusting or repulsive
Slimy	Despicable or worthless
Smelly	Stinking or reeking
Sobbing	Crying or weeping
Sorry	Apologetic or repentant
Spiteful	Vindictive or malicious
Sticky	Adhesive or delicate
Stinky	Malodorous or foul
Stormy	Turbulent or rough
Stressful	Worrying or exhausting
Stuck	Burdened or trapped
Stupid	Unintelligent or confused
Substandard	Inferior or unacceptable
Suspect	Questionable or doubtful
Suspicious	Distrustful or skeptical
Tearful	Crying or weeping
Tense	Uneasy or stressful

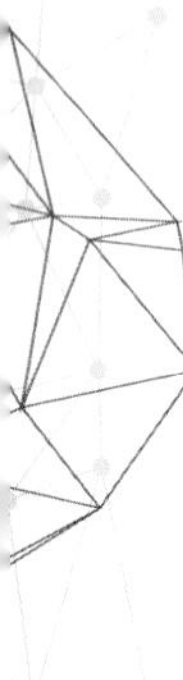

A to Z of negative words:	Meaning:
Terrible	Shocking or dreadful
Terrified	Frightened or panicky
Terrifying	Alarming or menacing
Threatening	Forbidding or intimidating
Unexpected	Unforeseen or surprising
Unfair	Unreasonable or discriminatory
Unfavorable	Negative or uncomplimentary
Unhappy	Miserable or despondent
Unhealthy	Unfit or poorly
Unlucky	Unfortunate or luckless
Unpleasant	Distressing or unpalatable
Unsatisfactory	Unacceptable or inadequate
Unwholesome	Harmful or unhealthy
Unwise	Foolish or irresponsible
Upset	Distressed, annoyed or worried
Vicious	Inhumane or savage
Wary	Suspicious or distrustful
Weary	Exhausted or fatigued
Windy	Blustery or squally
Worried	Troubled or tormented
Worthless	Meaningless or insignificant
Wound	Trauma or laceration
Yucky	Revolting or disgusting
Zero	Naught or nothing

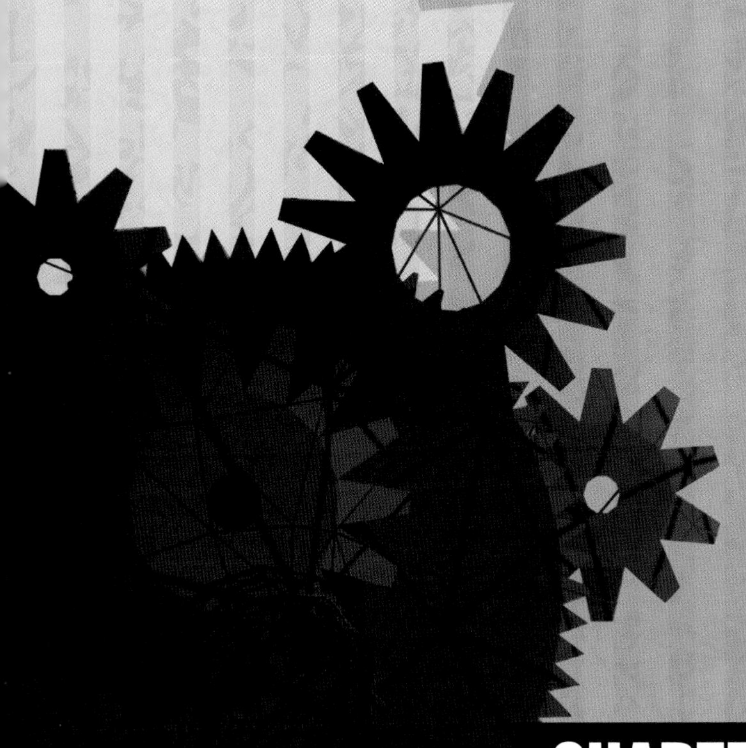

CHAPTER FOURTEEN.

CONCLUDING COMMENTS

FOURTEEN.

CONCLUDING COMMENTS

You should not be so engrossed with your mental thoughts or be in a trance-like mental state that you are unaware of what is going on around you when practicing mental rehearsal techniques during everyday life in training or when competing.

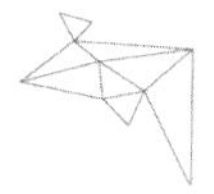

"Achieving happens with a series of events, first by thinking it, then saying it, then doing it." Mark Kleanthous

See you at the races!

For coaching and mentoring advice, contact

Mark Kleanthous

mark@ironmate.co.uk

www.ironmate.co.uk

Mark is also author of the *Complete Book of Triathlon Training* by Meyer and Meyer Sport.

ISBN 978-1-78255-022-8

Competitor of more than 460 triathlons, including 36 Ironman® double and triple Ironman® distance events.

When is the right time? Now is the time to start trying.

There are 86,400 seconds each and every day.

Don't wait for the perfect time, start today!

You have to create the perfect situation for the opportunity. When it happens you are ready.

If you are waiting for an opportunity you will fail because if that opportunity happens you will not be ready.

Don't be comfortable with the here and now.

Once you are satisfied you will start losing in life because you will never grow.

Get out of your comfort zone!

Overcome the enemy within and then you have overcome every enemy outside.

Spiritual suicide of the mind happens if you do not work day and night at your dreams and desires.

Make sacrifices to make your dreams become reality.

Reach high so you can keep growing, embrace the pain.

If it was easy everyone would do it.

You need motivation not to be a loser.

Increase the burning desire from within when life gets in the way of your ambition.

Do not let adversity get in your way.

When you stop wanting to achieve you will start to die in the mind.

Success comes from doing a lot of small things well.

Don't take your dreams to the graveyard!

CREDITS

Photos and graphics:

Coverphoto of Mark Kleanthous - Keith Greenlough

Page 8, Photo of Sean Conway - Martin Hartley

Page 69 - Thinkstock/Blend Images/Erik Isakson

Page 13, 29, 37, 87, 135, 139 - Thinkstock/Fuse

Molecule Graphic - Thinkstock/iStock/Godruma

Copyediting: Michelle Demeter

Coverdesign: Claudia Sakyi

Typesetting and Layout: Kristina Ehrhardt

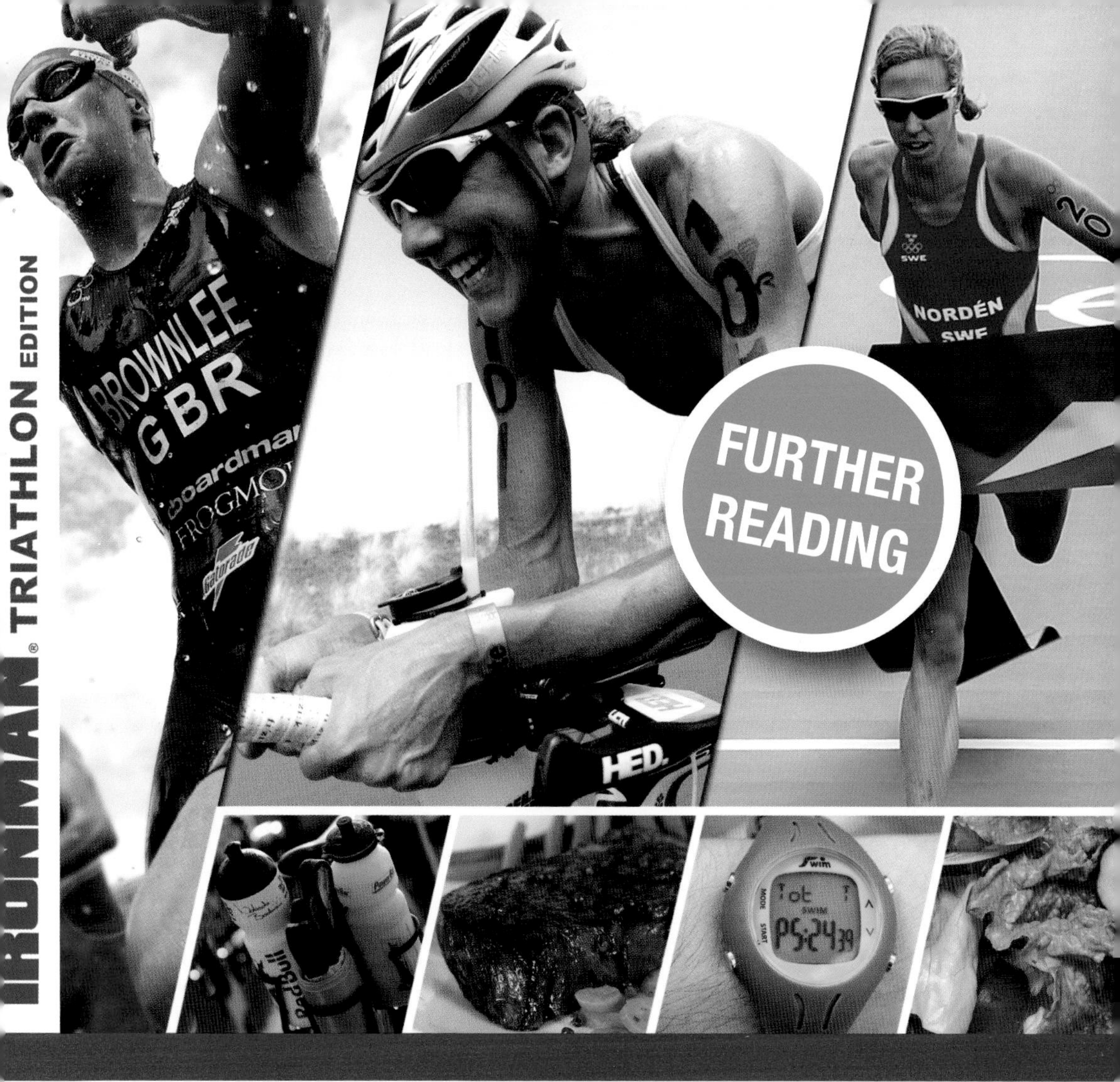

MARK KLEANTHOUS

THE COMPLETE BOOK OF TRIATHLON TRAINING

- PREPARING FOR A TRIATHLON COMPETITION
- TRAINING PLANS FOR ALL DISTANCES
- EQUIPMENT, DIET, NUTRITION & HYDRATION STRATEGY

THE ENCYCLOPEDIA OF TRIATHLON

MEYER & MEYER SPORT

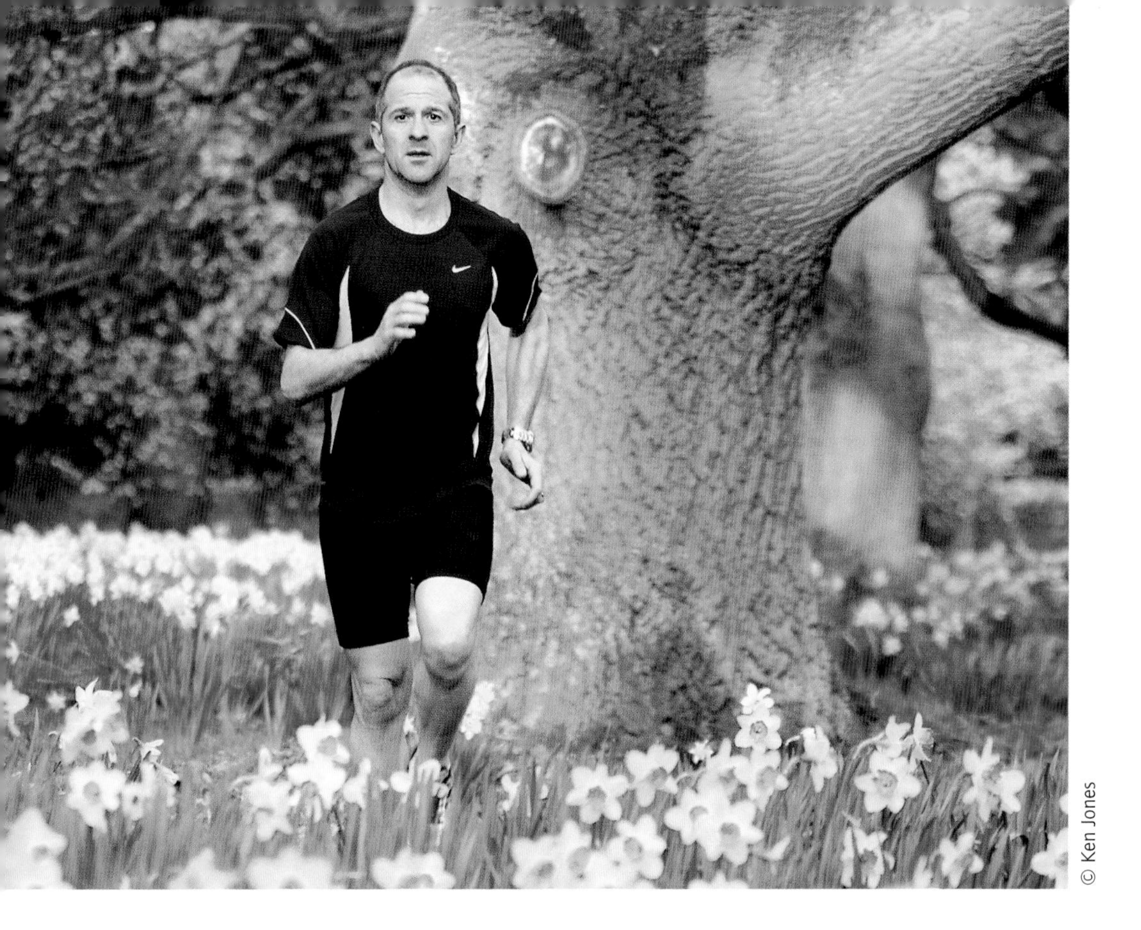

© Ken Jones

CHAPTER 5

The Theory of Training

If you are to devise an appropriate training session for yourself and apply it successfully, you will need to understand how that training will affect your body

THE FIVE FACTORS NECESSARY FOR TRIATHLON FITNESS

There are five main factors that contribute to fitness in triathlon – aerobic threshold endurance, nutrition, economy, strength, and recovery – but your approach to them has to be balanced. Neglect one and your performance will suffer.

I will now discuss each one of these in turn.

AEROBIC THRESHOLD ENDURANCE

The use of intense aerobic-threshold training (which, effectively, means training at your predicted triathlon pace) is perhaps the best way to get fit – the more you do, the easier the training session gets and the faster you become. But the problem is that we have a limited tolerance to this type of training, and the result can be overtraining. Therefore, not all your training should consist of intense, aerobic-threshold workouts.

This kind of training session is called a "key workout", and it is a common mistake to do too many of them with more than eight weeks to go before a triathlon. While there are many factors that can influence the amount you do, such as sporting background, age, sex, lifestyle, nutrition, sleep, non-active recovery, and stress levels to name just a few, my training ratio for athletes who work full-time is 28 weeks basic-endurance training then eight weeks building race-specific fitness. This way you will not experience burnout. In fact, you should only be tired for up to 36 hours after your key workouts. If you are permanently tired then you have other problems that need to be addressed, such as diet or the possibility that your workouts in between key sessions are too hard.

Because the triathlon is 140.6 miles long, it is very easy to train above the average triathlon pace all year long, as the triathlon marathon is likely to be 2min per mile slower than your fresh 10km pace. Training at your predicted triathlon pace will seem incredibly slow but that is what you need to do. It takes no more than eight weeks of anaerobic training to get race fit once you have developed a solid aerobic base. B and C races will provide you with more than enough aerobic-threshold training during your build up (see 'How to schedule progress', later in this chapter). Steady, even-paced endurance training allows you to recover while you race.

NUTRITION

In order to compete successfully in any long-distance event, you must be able to load your body with all the fuel necessary to propel yourself across the required distance at the desired speed. But this factor isn't only important when racing, because in order to complete your training successfully, your body must be constantly carrying the correct amount of fuel, and by that I mean the type of carbohydrates that can be accessed and fed to the muscles during the race.

In addition to this, you will need to either build up your body strength in certain areas or maintain the strength you already have, and that requires the continuous intake of a certain amount of protein. Developing a correct diet is as important as developing the right balance in training.

ECONOMY

Top triathletes all have one thing in common – they don't waste energy doing things they don't need to do. Anyone can load up their bodies with the required energy to complete the race, but if they then waste that energy because of an inefficient swimming, cycling or running style, they will usually be disappointed with the result.

Economy of movement is something that can be learnt early, so that it becomes a subconscious habit rather than something that needs to be constantly remembered.

STRENGTH

Strength is important in all sports, but athletes who are too bulky will never be successful in long-distance events. What is required is sport-specific strength to the level required, so that you don't carry too much weight into a race. All strength training therefore needs to be very carefully targeted toward specific muscles.

RECOVERY

Full-time athletes are obviously more successful than those who work full time because they can dedicate more time to training, but another, equally important reason is because they are able to take more recovery time.

I have no doubt that most injuries and illnesses are caused more by the lack of consistent sleep, regular massages, healthy food, stretches and cool downs than anything else. I call these double positives, because they not only help you recover from workouts, but more importantly they allow you to tolerate a greater amount of training. Fitness is about being able to recover as you train; the quicker the recovery, the greater the knock-on effect it has on fitness.

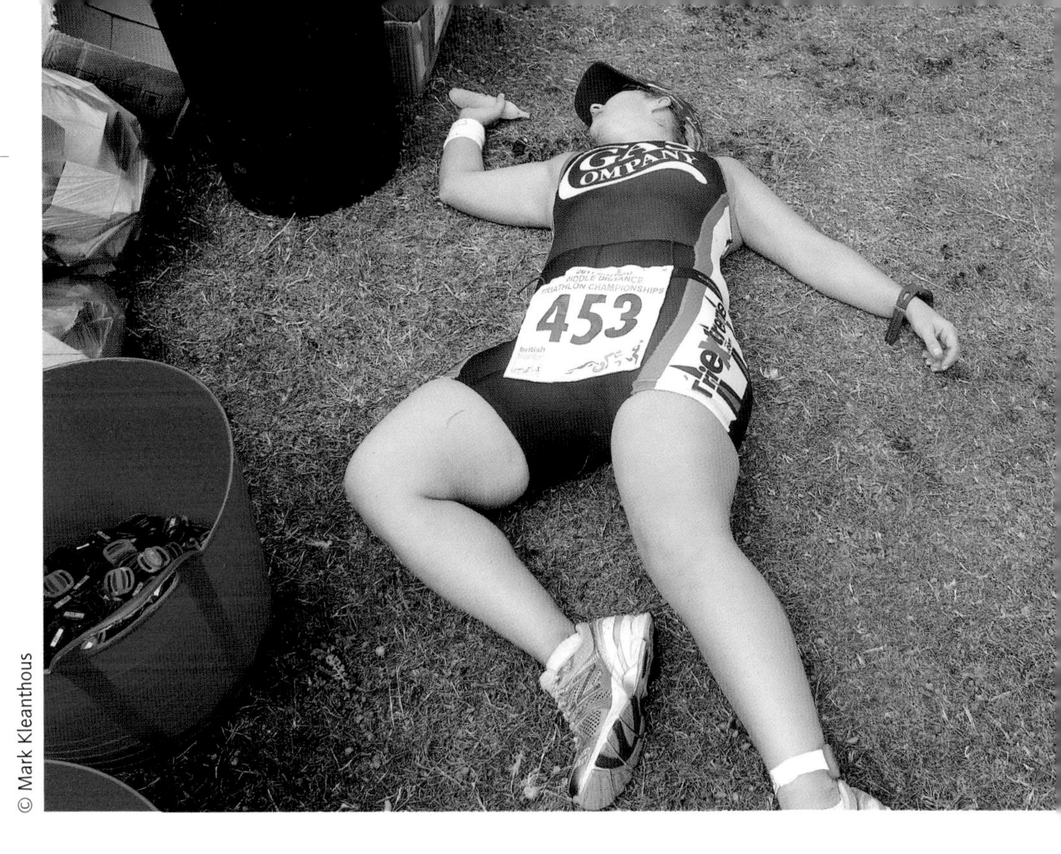

Every time you become fatigued, make a note of it, as that is your current ceiling for training. Recover correctly and your body will thank you by raising your ceiling to a higher level next time. Continued muscle soreness, lethargy or waves of sleepiness during the day are signs that you are doing too much.

TRAINING STRESS

As you begin training and your body starts to adapt to it, you will need to increase your effort just enough to improve but not so much that it has a harmful effect on your recovery, which would then reduce your performance. Improved performance comes from progressive training, and this is achieved by adding small amounts of training stress over time. Therefore, in order to be able to do this correctly, you will need to understand your own training stress levels. Without this information, you will only ever perform well during training, not on race day, as you will not be able to taper and peak – the keys to a good race performance.

Gradual increases in training stress levels (TSLs) can also increase fitness quicker than large increases. A sudden increase in the length of a run

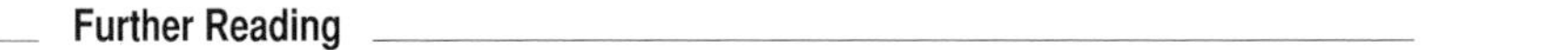

to 14 miles can give the body such a shock that the recovery time will be much longer than with two or three smaller increases spread over four weeks.

Once you have achieved your optimum training stress for a certain period of time, then any extra is not only useless, but it is actually detrimental to what you have already done. By understanding your personal training stress level, you will be able to plan a training programme that will allow you to improve and progress gradually without the peaks and troughs.

ISBN: 978-1-78255-022-8